The Complete Gay Divorce

The Complete
Gay Divorce

Brette McWhorter Sember,
Attorney At Law

CAREER
PRESS
Franklin Lakes, NJ

THE COMPLETE GAY DIVORCE
EDITED AND TYPESET BY GINA TALUCCI
Cover design by Mada Design, Inc.
Printed in the U.S.A. by Book-mart Press

To order this title, please call toll-free 1-800-CAREER-1 (NJ and Canada: 201-848-0310) to order using VISA or MasterCard, or for further information on books from Career Press.

CAREER
PRESS

The Career Press, Inc., 3 Tice Road, PO Box 687,
Franklin Lakes, NJ 07417
www.careerpress.com
www.newpagebooks.com
Library of Congress Cataloging-in-Publication Data

Sember, Brette McWhorter, 1968-
    The complete gay divorce / by Brett McWhorter Sember.
        p. cm.
    ISBN 1-56414-838-6 (paper)
        1. Same-sex divorce—United States. 2. Divorce settlements—United States. 3. Gay couples—Legal status, laws, etc. 4. Separation (psychology)—United States. I. Title.

HQ825.S45 2006
306.89086640973--dc22

                                                        2005053180

Acknowledgments

Many thanks to my wonderful agent, Gina Panettieri, for her wisdom and friendship, and to the terrific team at Career Press, including Michael Pye and Gina Talucci, for their vision and unflagging support. Special thanks go to Mike Lewis, Belle Wong, Brigitte Thompson, Tom and Kathleet McWhorter, and Megan Buckley. And as always, nothing would be possible without Terry, Quinne, and Zayne.

Contents

Introduction

Divorce is a big business in the United States. There are thousands of divorce attorneys, huge state systems set up to deal with the large volume of cases, marriage therapists, and more books than you can count about divorce. Yet somehow, gay and lesbian couples have been forgotten in all of this. Gays and lesbians commit to each other and have relationship failures like anyone else. They have children together. In some states, they marry. They share joint assets and joint debts. A gay divorce contains exactly the same elements as a heterosexual divorce, except no one seems to pay much attention to them.

If you're dealing with the end of a relationship, you're probably looking for answers. You're trying to figure out a way to take what was a completely conjoined life and turn it into two separate lives. You're looking for legal answers, emotional support, and, if you have children, ways to help them through this. You're going through a very difficult time and some support and information goes a long way toward helping you.

At the time this book was written, gay unions or marriage were legalized in three states (as well as in Canada, and overseas in Belgium, the Netherlands, and Spain), with other states allowing various kinds of partnerships. The tide is turning. Now that there are reasonable, legal ways to cement your life together, some couples will need reasonable, legal ways to undo their unions.

This book is your guide to the financial, legal, and practical aspects of the end of your relationship. Whether you filed a domestic partnership, were legally married or unioned, or have a committed relationship that is not recognized by your state, you are going through a divorce. You are separating from your life partner and unraveling the threads that hold you together. Doing this can be quite confusing when you try to navigate custody, child support, joint property, joint debts, or a need for spousal support after your relationship ends. All the answers you need are in this book. Solutions for every kind of long-term relationship breakup are included. You'll not only find information on state laws and procedures, but suggestions on how to divide things, help your children, and get yourself through this difficult time.

Keep in mind that this book is as up to date as possible, but this is a rapidly developing area of law with frequent changes. It's always best to check with an attorney in your state so that you can understand your state's laws and your rights.

The book refererences many Websites where you can get more information. Website addresses are constantly changing, so if any do not work, go to the home page for that site and see if you can locate the information you need from there.

Throughout this book, I will use the word "divorce" to refer to any relationship that is ending, whether or not you are eligible for an actual legal divorce.

This publication is designed to provide accurate and authoritative information in regard to the subject matter covered. It is sold with the understanding that the publisher or author is not engaged in rendering legal, accounting, or other professional service. If legal advice or other expert assistance is required, the services of a competent professional person should be sought. This book is not a substitute for legal advice.

The process you're facing is not an easy one, but you will get through it and move on with your life. Focus on the future as you work through the challenges facing you today, and remember that this is only one short stage in your life. It *will* get better.

Chapter 1

Deciding to Divorce

The decision to end a relationship is a very painful one and isn't one that can be made lightly. When you and your partner committed to each other, got a civil union, or got married, you did so intending to spend the rest of your lives together. Seeing that come to an end is probably one of the most difficult situations you'll face in your life.

This is a tough time for you. Not only are you facing emotional turmoil and pain, but you are faced with complicated choices when it comes to your legal options. You have many decisions to make and a lot to think about. But you can get through it all and you will be okay. The best way to start coping is to keep your eyes firmly focused on the future and your heart centered on the belief that you will find happiness once the separation is over. Make decisions one at a time and give yourself time and space to work through them.

Is Your Relationship Over?

It can be hard to tell if you have problems that can be fixed or if you need to call it quits. Sometimes it's immediately clear if a relationship is over, but most of the time there are opportunities to work out your problems. Ending your relationship should be a careful decision and one that you give some time to. Divorce is a gradual process that actually begins long before you actively think about ending the relationship. It is a slow pulling apart that eventually creates a rift that won't heal.

If you're undecided about whether a divorce or break up really is the best solution, ask yourself:

▼ Do my spouse and I have the same level of commitment to our relationship?

▼ Does my partner make me feel happy, secure, loved, and valued?

▼ Why are we staying together?

▼ Do we fight constantly?

▼ How will I feel if I am alone?

▼ How will a break up affect our children?

▼ Can I survive financially on my own?

▼ Do I feel resentment and contempt?

▼ Do we avoid spending time together?

▼ Am I happy right now?

▼ Where do I want to be in five years?

▼ Has our physical relationship changed?

▼ Has one of us broken a promise of sexual fidelity?

▼ Does one or both of us want to see other people?

▼ Do we have a lack of respect for each other?

You might also try making a pro and con list. List reasons why you should stay and reasons why you should leave, and see which side of the list is more convincing. Talking to yourself is another way to help make this decision. Research has shown that people who talk out loud to themselves when they are in a crisis tend to make better decisions. Talking stimulates other areas of your brain, and can help you work through options.

Don't give yourself deadlines. Saying, "I have to make a decision about this by Monday," is not helpful. When the time is right, you'll know.

Some couples decide on a trial separation to find out if they really want to be apart. Although this might be painful, it can be a helpful way to really see if you want to stay together. Living in a divorced or separated situation can be very different from what you imagine. You can learn a lot about yourself and your relationship if you take a break. Some therapists recommend that you mentally live with the decision to divorce for one week (even if you still live together) so that you can see what it feels like emotionally.

Getting Help to Save Your Relationship

Even if you're not ready to walk away, you're probably certain that there are some serious issues in your relationship that need to be resolved. If you've gotten to the point of considering a divorce or split, then the problems you're facing are pretty serious. It's unlikely that they're going to go away by themselves. So, if you really want to continue the relationship, consider getting help from a mental health professional. It might seem difficult to find a therapist who is experienced in gay relationships, but they do exist. These resources listed on the following page can help find someone near you:

▼ Gay and Lesbian International Therapist Search Engine *www.glitse.com.*

▼ Gay and Lesbian National Hotline THE-888-GLNH.

▼ American Association for Marriage and Family Therapy (202) 452-0109 or *www.aamft.org.*

A therapist can help you find new ways to look at certain areas of your life and help change your behavior. Therapy is hard work though, and if you're going to try it, you must truly commit to make it work the way it is supposed to. If you walk in thinking it's not going to be successful, then it won't. If you feel there is anything in your relationship worth salvaging, therapy is the way to make that rescue.

❖Kathleen and Beth have been together for 24 years and have twice been on the verge of breaking up. They found a lesbian counselor using a gay community directory and counseled with her for almost a year about issues such as power and control, sharing their living space, and how changes in their work impacted their relationship. Several years later, they returned to counseling for a few months to get some more help as changes happened in their lives. Counseling saved their relationship.

Divorce and Children

Many people believe that if you have children, staying together for their sake is the best option. A divorce or breakup does have an impact on children, but I always told my clients that dealing with divorced parents is much better than dealing with parents who always fight. Living in a home where there is screaming, yelling, and a lack of love and respect is far more damaging than having two parents living happily in separate homes. The decision to separate or divorce has to be one that you make based on your own needs and situation. Your children are a big part of your situation, so you *should* take their needs into account, but they should not be the determining factor. You have to decide what is best for you and your family overall.

Even if your children are not legally related to both of you, the divorce will have an impact on them. Suddenly a person that has filled a parental role on a daily basis will be gone from the child's life. When you're making the decision whether or not to divorce or separate you should not discuss this decision with your kids. The appropriate time to talk to your kids is after you have made a decision and have some kind of plan in place. It is always best if you and your spouse or partner can sit down and explain it to your child together. The decision to divorce or break up must be made by the two adults who created the relationship and the family. See Chapter 10 for more information about how breakups affect children.

> ❖David and Peter had been together for nine years and had a 6 year old son. Peter was desperately unhappy, but terrified to break up their family. He was sure that if they split, their son would grow up dysfunctional. Even before the potential breakup, the son had problems with authority and difficulty sleeping. It's hard enough to be the child of gay parents, but to be the child of gay parents who are no longer together seemed an impossible situation to Peter. David and Peter finally did separate and now live within several blocks of each other.
> *continued on next page*

Their son spends time with both of them and their new partners. He's currently 9 years old and plays soccer, does well in school, and has solid friendships. Looking back on it, Peter says, "Splitting up was really the best decision. I was afraid of what kind of effect it would have on him, but really he adjusted beautifully to the break up. We still parent together and we are both completely there for him. He has two loving parents, two loving stepparents, and he doesn't have to hide under the covers like he used to when he heard us screaming at each other. If we had stayed together we would have both been miserable and I know he would have been, too. It was a bad situation and now he's living in a good situation."

Temporary Court Orders

Once you've made the decision to part ways, there are a variety of legal options available to you that will be discussed later in this book. While you consider your long-term options, it's important to know that there are some short-term solutions that can help you now.

The best way to deal with interim decisions is to make them yourselves. Work out separate plans for how you are going to deal with money, time with the kids, and living arrangements while you are working through your divorce or breakup.

If you have children together and cannot agree on a temporary arrangement, you can obtain a temporary court order directing custody, visitation, and child support from your local family court which will stay in place until you make final decisions. If you and your partner are the legal parents of the child, you are entitled to seek intervention from the court regardless of whether you are married or not. A temporary order can calm everyone down and lay out some basic rules so you can organize your lives and make sure your child is cared for and is not in the middle of a tug of war. It takes care of the immediate crisis and the disagreement you are having for the time being and allows everyone time to think.

If you live in Vermont, Connecticut, or Massachusetts and were married or unioned under those state's laws, you can also seek a temporary order of spousal support, which can help you survive financially when you've just broken up and haven't had time to file for a divorce yet.

You can go to your local family court and file the papers yourself or, you can hire an attorney to do so for you. Most family courts are user-friendly and will assist you in completing paperwork to get a temporary order.

Coming to Terms With What You Want

It's one thing to decide you want a divorce or separation, but it's another to face the very detailed decisions you will need to make about dividing belongings and financial matters. Whether you are legally married or without any formal agreement, you have the absolute right to some of the belongings and property you obtained together during your relationship and to some of your joint funds. You have the absolute right to seek custody or visitation with any child you are legally related to and to seek child support. You have the right to a fair division of your joint debts. These are your rights, but you need to think carefully about what you really want.

A divorce or breakup is not just about material possessions, and focusing too much on this aspect can really make you crazy. Your self-worth is not (or should not be) tied up in whether you get the baker's rack and the Dansk place settings. You must decide how you want to come out of this process emotionally. Some people really just want closure. Other people have an ax to grind or a point to make. You've got to work through your feelings at your own pace and in your own way and come to your own conclusions about what is important to you. You must decide what kind of divorce you want and also consider what kind of divorce your partner is going to make it into. If you want it to be amicable and he or she wants total war, it's unlikely you're going to be able to make it amicable.

It's important to be realistic about divorce. Some people assume the worst and see divorce as a knock down, drag out fight. It doesn't have to be that way. Other people think they can sort things out on their own, shake hands, and wish each other well. They are surprised to find that there really is a lot of emotion involved and it's difficult to turn it all off. There is a happy medium though, and you can treat each other decently and still work out an agreement that gives both of you most of what you want, while dealing with the emotional upheavals.

You and your partner should consider setting up some ground rules to help you get through the divorce process. Some examples include:

▼ Agree not to scream and yell at each other.

▼ Focus on the issues that are in front of you and try not to tie them into past events or problems.

▼ Be fair to each other.

▼ If you haven't physically separated yet, give each other time and space.

▼ Try not to use guilt as a weapon.

▼ Try not to be vengeful or do things you know will hurt the other person just because you can.

▼ Come up with a signal, such as "time out" that means you both need to step away and cool down before going any further.

▼ Agree that you will not use your children as bargaining chips and will not try to get them involved in the adult decisions you will be making.

▼ Decide to try to deal with money in a way that is fair and leaves each partner financially stable.

Think about how you're going to manage your divorce by answering the following questions:

▼ Describe how you want your divorce to go.

▼ Describe how you think your partner wants it to go.

▼ Describe what you can do together to make this process go as smoothly as possible and to make it as emotionally manageable as possible.

Now that you've considered the big picture, it's time to begin to think about some of the details. Taking some time to think now about what you really want out of your divorce will help you make decisions as you move through each step in the process.

▼ Do you want custody or visitation with your child? Describe what kind of arrangement you want.

▼ Do you want ownership of a home, vehicle, or other large item of property?

▼ Do you want a cash settlement? Describe what you think is fair.

▼ Do you want to continue to receive health insurance benefits through your partner or spouse?

▼ Do you need financial support after the separation to help you get on your feet, get a job, or get an education? Describe how much you need.

▼ Create a list of the most important items of joint property (things you acquired together during your relationship) that you want to have.

Later, you'll find chapters in the book that will help you work through each category and hammer out the details, but now you've set some basic goals. Don't be surprised if you goals change as you work through the divorce process. Your goals will be constantly evolving. You are in a period of great change right now and you can't expect to know exactly where you're going.

Finding the Courage to Ask for What You Need

Now that you've thought out what you want to walk out of the marriage or relationship with, it's time to think about putting yourself in a position to ask for those things. You have the right to ask for all of the things you just described. It doesn't matter whether your state recognizes your relationship or not. In some states, you can go to court and ask for the things you described. In states where you can't do this, you can still work out a divorce arrangement with your partner. In every state, if you have joint assets, there is legal assistance available to sort it out.

You have the right to stand up as a person and end your relationship in a way that works for you, is comfortable for you, and takes care of your needs. But you must find the courage and the strength to ask for what you need.

Staying Safe

Domestic violence happens in both gay and straight couples across the board and anyone who experiences it deserves help and support. Unfortunately there is a lack of awareness about gay domestic violence. Domestic violence shelters may not be willing to accept gay men who are seeking protection, because the victims that the shelters focus on are mostly women. (Regardless of this, you should always contact them if you need help and they may be able to suggest some other kind of assistance in your area.) You are always entitled to legal and police protection if you are in danger from your partner.

If you experience domestic violence you must first worry about your safety and that of your children before anything else. Get out of the house and get away from the abuser as quickly as possible. Call 911 if you are in danger. Don't let any police officer think you're not serious. You have the right to police assistance.

For help, assistance, information, and support contact:

▼ Rainbow Domestic Violence
   www.rainbowdomesticviolence.itgo.com.

▼ National Domestic Violence Hotline
   (800) 799-7233.

▼ Gay on Gay Violence:
   www.web.apc.org/~jharnick/violence.html.

▼ The Network:
   www.thenetworklared.org/ or call their hotline
   at (617) 423-SAFE.

You are entitled to seek a protective order from your
local family or criminal court if you believe you are in
danger from your spouse or partner. No one can stop you
from asking the court for protection. You can go to your
local family court and ask for help filing the papers. If you
contact the police, they will help you file a complaint. Your
area may have a victim's support team that will assign a
volunteer to support you when you go to court or have to
talk to police or attorneys. If you need help, ask. No one
will know what you are going through and what you need
if you do not speak up.

Gay males in abusive relationships have one of the highest
incidences of drug abuse. If you or your partner has a
drug problem, get help. These organizations can help you
get assistance:

▼ National Drug & Alcohol Treatment Hotline:
   (800) 662-HELP.

▼ American Council on Alcoholism: (800) 527-5344.

▼ National Clearinghouse for Alcohol and Drug
   Information: (800) 729-6686.

▼ National Council on Alcoholism and Drug
   Dependence: (800) 622-2255.

▼ National Council on Alcohol and Drugs: (800) 475-HOPE.

▼ Gay and Lesbian National Hotline: (888) 843-4564.

❖Susan was in an abusive lesbian relationship. It took her a long time to realize that she deserved better and that she could make it on her own. She started secretly seeing a therapist who encouraged her to leave and helped her understand that she was not to blame for the abuse. When she was ready to leave, the therapist was able to contact a local shelter for her and make arrangements for her to go there. She went to court and got an order of protection against her partner. She later realized how lucky she was to have gotten out safely and to have had a therapist who helped her through the decision.

Chapter 2

The Divorce or Breakup Process

When your relationship ends, it's a divorce whether or not your state recognizes it. When you are married in your hearts, you go through the same emotional steps a couple married in the eyes of the law goes through. The label for what you're going through doesn't change the impact it has on your personal life. Understanding the common steps people in a divorce go through can help you see where you're going and what you will be dealing with.

The Three Types of Divorce

When you divorce, there are several important levels on which you experience the break up, all of which are equally difficult.

Emotional Divorce

The first type of divorce is the emotional divorce. This is where you decide together, or come to realize by yourself, that your relationship is over or that you no longer love or want to be with each other. This realization is the one that starts the breakup and can be a long and involved process stretching months or even years. Whether this is something you've been mulling over for some time or it is something that has come as a sudden shock, it is equally difficult and painful. It's important to note that couples spend a lot of time in limbo over this decision. One day you might be certain you want to break up, while other days you feel scared and unsure. It's okay to take time to come to a decision.

Coping with the emotional divorce is the most difficult part of the situation you are facing and it is important to realize that it is a lengthy process. You won't suddenly wake up tomorrow, next week, or even next month and decide that you're over it. You will probably go through many ups and downs. Some days will be easier than others and you must give yourself time. Depending on what kind of legal process you have to deal with, your divorce could last more than a year. If you are going through a court divorce you will have ups and downs and lots of frustrations to deal with. It's important to remember that you will get through it and you will come out the other side ready to move on with your life.

It is also important that you allow no one to undermine what you are experiencing. You are going through a divorce, whether or not your state labels it as such. Unfortunately there are still many people who fail to understand that your break up is just as devastating as any heterosexual divorce. It may help if you use the word *divorce*. (New terms that have recently been coined are the words *givorce* or *gayvorce* used to refer to gay break ups or the end of a civil union or domestic partnership) when talking about your situation. This can help drive home what's really going on.

It is important to get support from people who love you and understand your pain. Family and friends may provide this for you. You may also find that a good therapist is worth his or her weight in gold, as you work through the sadness of the end of your relationship. See Chapter 14 for more help on obtaining closure and support.

Physical Divorce

The physical divorce is your actual physical separation from each other. For some couples this happens immediately when one moves out. For others, this may be more time-consuming, particularly if there are legal issues to resolve about finances. Sometimes a couple will remain in the same home, but live in separate rooms until all the details of their separation have been worked out.

You and your partner must do what works best for you. If an immediate physical separation will give you room to breathe or time to think, then make it a priority. If, however, you don't find your current situation unbearable, avoiding immediate rash decisions can be helpful as you try to sort out the conjoined property and finances you have together. It's important to remember that if you are dealing with children, the physical separation will have a huge impact on them, and also probably on your custody case, if it will be going to court. Moving out of a home you partly own also may hurt your chances of getting ownership of it, so these are important considerations to keep in mind when thinking about a physical separation.

For some people, physically separating is an extremely difficult hurdle, while for others it is a relief. Remember that there is no one right answer and that you must do what works best in your individual situation.

Legal or Practical Divorce

Depending on where you live or where you were married, you may or may not have a legal divorce on your hands. (See Chapters 3 and 4.) But even so, you do have a practical divorce to go through. This involves dissolving any legal ties between the two of you including: joint accounts, a jointly owned or leased home, dividing personal property, and undoing any legal unions or marriages.

The best way to cope with the practical divorce is to take things one step at a time. For example, it can be overwhelming to look at all the belongings you've got to go through and divide into two piles, but if you take things slowly and try not to let yourself get overwhelmed, you will get through the process.

The most important thing to remember about the practical divorce is to try and approach it in a rational and careful way. Of course you're upset and you don't know which way is up, but if you let your emotions guide you, you may make mistakes that you will later regret. Give yourselves time to work through the decisions facing you. You can't do this in one afternoon and you shouldn't feel pressured to rush through it.

If you are going through a court process, expect that it will last longer than you assume. Court schedules and attorneys are busy and even if you're ready to move forward, your case will probably take much longer than you think. It's easy to let a court divorce make you crazy. The entire process seems to be geared towards making you hate, and want to hurt each other. Fortunately there are other alternatives you can use, such as reaching a settlement on your own or using mediation (see Chapter 13), which are much easier emotionally and will help resolve things much faster.

Issues in a Divorce

When your relationship ends there are several types of issues you have to consider and work through. These are things that concern you whether you are legally married or not, because they are decisions you can make even if the law does not support them in your state. The decisions in a divorce include the following:

Parenting

If you or your partner have children who were part of your life together, you will have to make decisions about this. If you are legal parents together, your state family court will address issues of custody and visitation if you cannot reach an agreement, but if you both are not legal parents, you can still create a plan together to keep both of you in your child's life. Parenting is one of the most important decisions you will make in your divorce and this decision will have an impact on all of your other decisions. For example, who keeps the house and how you divide up belongings is impacted by who the child will mainly live with. It is often helpful to try to talk and think about your parenting decisions before you deal with the other issues facing you. If you can come up with a solid parenting plan, it may allow all the other decisions to logically fall into place. See Chapter 10 for more information about parenting.

Child Support

If you are legal parents together, your state support laws will apply to your situation and one of you will pay child support to the other. You can create a child support agreement, but it will have to be approved by the court (because it must meet minimum levels set up by your state).

If you are not legal parents together, it is still possible for you to discuss some kind of informal support arrangement if this is what you both want. See Chapter 11 for more information about child support.

Property Division

Most couples have some kind of joint property, be it real estate, cars, boats, household items, bank accounts, or investments. Dividing up these joint assets can be a difficult and time-consuming process. If your marriage was a legal one your state will have laws governing how you do this, but you are able to create a settlement as long as it is fair. If your marriage was not legally recognized, you have the freedom to divide property in any way you wish, but you may have the problem of not being able to agree how to go about this.

You also may have joint debts, or debts that you feel jointly responsible for even though they may be in one person's name. You'll need to make decisions about how you will divide responsibility for these debts. See Chapter 11 for more information about property and debt division.

Financial Support

Spousal support, or alimony, is another option open to you and your partner. Alimony can help one partner get back onto his or her feet financially after a breakup and, even if you are not legally married, you can create an arrangement to do this. See Chapter 12 for more information about alimony.

Type of Legal Process to Use

You must also decide what, if any, legal process you are going to use to end your marriage. For example, if you were civil unioned in Vermont, but live in Florida, it may be too much of a burden on you to go back to Vermont to get a divorce. You and your partner must decide what there is to undo and if you want to take the time and money to undo it in the eyes of the law. This can be a very difficult and symbolic decision. It is also a decision that has future implications for both of you. Right now it might not seem to matter whether you dissolve your civil union, but if you want to remarry in the future, you will be unable to do so unless you dissolve your civil union at some point. Also, if gay marriage does become more widespread and more states recognize it (or even the federal government) your undissolved union could become important and affect your tax status in the future. It is also important to keep in mind that it may be easier to take the legal steps to dissolve a union now than it would be to track your partner down in 10 years and get it done then.

Annulment vs. Divorce

If you are eligible for a legal divorce, you may also be eligible for a legal annulment. An annulment is a decision by a court saying that your marriage was never valid in the first place. If one of you was underage, you are related to each other, one of you was coerced to marry, or one of you lied to the other about an important fact (such as whether you have a child), you may be eligible for an annulment. An annulment reverses the marriage and says that legally, it never existed in the first place. Children born or adopted into a marriage are still considered legitimate and legal children of both parents even if the marriage is annulled. Annulments are usually done with marriages of short duration and often there is little to decide in the way of property settlements. The procedure for an annulment is identical to that of a divorce in most states. Some people prefer an annulment when possible because it has a more positive sound to it. If you want an annulment, you need an attorney to represent you.

Grounds

When you ask for a divorce or dissolution, if you are eligible for one, you must offer a reason why you are seeking a formal end to the relationship. There are two types of reasons. A no-fault divorce means that you are able to tell the court you're both seeking the divorce and are not pointing fingers at each other. You agree that there has been a breakdown in your relationship that can't be repaired and you aren't required to provide more details. A fault divorce means that one of you must formally blame the other for the divorce. The terms could be abandonment, adultery, being in jail during the marriage, or because he or she treated you cruelly. If the other partner does not consent to the divorce, you have to have a grounds trial and prove your reason. It can get quite ugly, even if the other spouse consents to the divorce. Once you introduce an element of blame into the divorce, you can never repair the damage that it does. If you are confronted with a choice about a fault or no-fault divorce, choosing a no-fault divorce is always easier and better for everyone.

Prenuptial Agreements

If you and your partner entered into a prenuptial agreement and were legally married or unioned, the terms of that agreement will be followed in determining the terms of your divorce (assuming the prenup is valid). If you entered into what you think of as a prenup, but never legally married, see Chapter 5 about domestic partnership contracts.

Court Procedures

Each state has different procedures, forms, and rules when it comes to divorce, dissolution of civil unions or domestic partnerships, or court proceedings for custody or child support. Later in this book we will discuss the forms for divorce or dissolution in the states that offer them. If you will be going to court for custody or child support, you need to get the right forms for your state (usually easily available at your local family courthouse, or on your state judiciary Website).

Court procedures vary widely, but there are some similarities. In most cases you will file an initial paper with the court that begins whatever kind of case you are starting. This is sometimes called a complaint or petition. Usually there is an initial appearance where the court simply verifies things and schedules a later date. There is often a period of time for attorneys to gather evidence. This is called discovery. Most courts hold pretrial conferences in which the parties are encouraged to find a settlement. Trials can volved in your case.

There are many elements that can help make your day in court a lot easier and less stressful. The following is a list of tips that can help you deal with court apperances:

▼ Dress conservatively. This means no piercings, relatively flat hair, little jewelry, no sandals or flip flops, and clothing that includes dress shirts, nice pants, possibly a tie or sport coat for men, and a dress, pant suit, skirt and top, or pants and nice top for women.

▼ Do not bring your child or children with you unless you are asked to do so by the judge or your attorney.

▼ Do not bring food, beverages, or gum.

▼ Turn off your cell phone before you enter the building.

▼ Refer to the judge as "Your Honor." Sir or ma'am is also acceptable.

▼ Be polite to court personnel. They can be a big help to you.

▼ Avoid getting into any kind of confrontation with your partner while in the building. If you have to, avoid all contact while in the waiting room. Do not speak to your partner in the courtroom. You are both speaking only to the judge and your own attorneys.

▼ Be patient. Some courts have long waits. You also need to realize that things won't be resolved on your first or second trips there. Divorce or custody proceedings can take months.

▼ If you cannot afford an attorney, but would like one, let the court personnel and the judge know. Your state or county may have a free legal services program that you are eligible for.

▼ Don't worry about being emotional. The end of a marriage or family is a very difficult time and everyone there understands what you're experiencing.

▼ Do bring along a friend or support person, but understand he or she may be not allowed to enter the courtroom.

▼ Be prepared to go through a metal detector and leave anything at home that might be construed as a weapon (including pocket knives).

▼ Show up at your appointed time. If you can't come for some reason, you must call your attorney (if you have one) or the court clerk in advance and let them know the reason for your absence. If you simply don't show up, the case can be heard without your input.

▼ Assume that you will get nothing but respect from the court personnel, attorneys, and judge involved in your case. This may not always be the reality of the situation, but if you act as if you deserve respect, it goes a long way towards adjusting how people treat you.

If you live in a state where marriage, civil union, or domestic partnership is available, but you and your partner have not taken advantage of this benefit and are now breaking up, you're going to find that the laws governing the breakup of those relationships don't apply to you because you don't have that piece of paper. You'll be left to negotiate an end to your partnership on your own, or through mediation. Some couples who find themselves in this situation might want to consider going and getting the piece of paper (marriage certificate, civil union certificate, or domestic partnership registration) and then turn around and go through the process to dissolve it soon after in order to give themselves access to the legal system. If you and your partner are in agreement or think you will be able to reach a settlement, there is no benefit to doing this (and it would simply add extra steps and expenses), but there are some couples who really need the structure of a legal procedure to help guide them through the breakup process, and for these couples, this rather unusual solution might be the right answer.

Legal Effect

If you obtain a divorce, the divorce itself is not recognized in other states, but any provisions of your divorce order, or any other family court order you obtain about custody and child support will be upheld by any state because custody and child support laws are almost universally recognized and respected from state to state. So if you have problems with visitation or child support, you can seek help from your home state court by showing your court order.

Getting Help

In later chapters dealing with specific states, you will find contact information for lawyer referral programs in those states, as well as whatever self-help legal information the states make available. All states have lawyer referral programs, so contact your state or local bar association for a referral to an attorney who can help you with your case. The American Academy of Matrimonial Lawyers can also refer you to an attorney in any state. Use the online search directory at *www.aaml.org/Directory.htm* and just type in the state you need. AAML attorneys must certify that they are experienced in matrimonial cases before they are permitted to join, so you can be certain that any attorney you are referred to is a specialist in this area. This does not mean, however, that he or she has any experience with same sex marriage, so be sure to ask when interviewing attorneys.

You may also be able to locate an attorney by talking to friends, or checking your local alternative or gay phone book (sometimes called The Lavender Pages) or by reading the ads and sponsors in local GLBT publications such as magazines, newspapers, or programs for community events or performances.

After you get some names of attorneys, set up free consultations with each one (either by phone or in person). See the questions later in this chapter that you should ask when interviewing the attorney.

If you cannot afford an attorney and you live in a state where your marriage is legally recognized, you may be able to obtain free or low cost legal help from a local legal aid office (check your phone book or call the local bar association). It is also possible to ask the court to direct your spouse to pay your attorney fees. If you want to try to do this, you need to find an attorney who agrees to this arrangement and can ask the court for this.

If you live in a state where your marriage is not recognized, or you were never married or unioned, you may be able to obtain free legal help for custody and child support cases through legal aid or a public defenders office.

When looking for an attorney to represent you, there are many things that should be considered before you decide on someone who is right for you and your particular situation. The following is a list of questions that can be helpful in the search for assistance:

▼ Are you gay? Do you consider yourself gay-friendly? Is your staff gay-friendly?

▼ What are your fees? Is there a nonrefundable retainer? What is your hourly rate? Does it increase for in-court time? What is the total estimate for the cost of this case? Are there court fees in addition to your fees?

▼ Do I need to sign a retainer agreement with you?

▼ What is your experience handling this kind of case? How many have you handled? How many have you won?

▼ How often should I expect to hear from you during the course of my case?

▼   Do you have a policy about how quickly you or your staff returns phone calls from clients?

▼   Do you believe mediation is a viable option in this case? Can you recommend a mediator to help us?

▼   How long do you expect this case to take?

▼   What are my chances of getting what I'm asking for in the divorce?

▼   Do you feel I am being reasonable in what I am seeking? Would you recommend I ask for anything else?

▼   How do the courts in our state rule on the issues in my case? Are there certain guidelines or precedents I should be aware of?

▼   What is my next step if I want to work with you?

▼   How soon can you begin this case?

▼   Is there anything I should do or not do with regard to my ex?

When You First Separate

When one of you moves out, it is a difficult and painful time, however this is a time when you need to keep your wits about you and keep your best interests in mind. Make sure, whether you move out or your partner moves out, that you have your birth certificate, passport, credit cards and ATM card, originals or copies of all financial documents, documents pertaining to your children if they will be living with you, your will, powers of attorney, health care directive or living will, title and all keys to your car, insurance policies and health insurance card and stocks or bonds belonging to you.

If you and your spouse have joint bank accounts, either one of you can access and remove all the funds in the account. Withdraw the money and divide it up. Or if you have not yet agreed on how to divide it, you can remove it yourself and place it in an individual account and hold it until you reach an agreement.

Put a freeze on all joint credit cards, or your cards on which your partner is an authorized user. You don't want to rack up any further joint debt or have your partner incur any further debt on your card. Open individual accounts and use those from now on.

Change your passwords on all of your accounts and online accounts. If your partner has moved out, you may want to change the locks on your home and move where you hide your key.

If things between you and your partner are very unpleasant you may also want to keep an eye on your mail to be sure things aren't missing. If they are, or you are worried about this, get a P.O. Box.

> ❖ Lindsey no longer loved Toni, but Toni seemed unable to let go of the relationship. Even after Lindsey moved out, Toni called her, stopped by her apartment, and even sent her mail at work. The final straw was when Lindsey came down to get her car one day only to find it was gone. Toni still had the extra keys. Lindsey realized that there were a lot of things she had not done to protect herself, such as changing her passwords and keeping an eye on her mail. A mutual friend later convinced Toni to give the car back and Lindsey took steps to keep Toni from interfering with her life. Lindsey now thinks that she was too trusting and naïve, and wishes she had understood that protecting herself should have been her first priority.

Making Decisions

Looking at all the various decisions you have to make can be mind-boggling. Use these tips to help you work through the choices you will be making:

▼ Remember that the average heterosexual divorce takes at least one year from start to finish, so give yourselves some time to make the decisions.

▼ Think about where you're both going and what you're both doing. Base decisions on your plans for your separate lives.

▼ Get help when you need it. There are many excellent therapists who can help you with the emotional part of your divorce. There are also a growing number of lawyers versed in this area of law who can help you with the legal issues.

▼ Approach things in an organized fashion. Gather all the documents and papers about joint assets and debts and keep them in an accordion file or plastic box so you can access them easily. It may be helpful to make lists of things you need to divide or things you need to decide about.

▼ If you will be pursuing any kind of legal dissolution to your relationship, start a file now where you can keep all documents and correspondence about this.

▼ Remember that neither one of you are going to walk away from this whole, complete, and untouched. You will both be affected financially and emotionally, and your home life will be disrupted.

▼   There are some decisions that can only be
made after others have been decided. Follow
the natural order of what needs to be decided
first. Parenting issues are usually of primary
importance. Living arrangements are usually
next in line. Decisions about asset and debt
division precede decisions about spousal
support.

Negotiating Decisions

The best way to make decisions with your partner about
your divorce is through negotiation. If you are legally joined,
you have a legal process available to you, if you choose, to
resolve the issues you're confronting. But if you have no
legal process to rely on, or believe that the decisions about
the end of your relationship are best made by the two of
you and not a court, negotiation is the best plan.

You and your partner can sit down and work through
the issues and options discussed in this book. The key word
in negotiation is *compromise*. Your relationship was a give
and take, and its dissolution must be as well.

To have a successful negotiation session, factor in these
suggestions:

▼   **Set ground rules.** Decide in advance how long
you will meet for and what you will be discussing. Create boundaries, such as no yelling,
pushing of hot buttons, or discussion of what
went wrong in the relationship.

▼   **Keep your kids out of it.** Don't try to negotiate
or work things out in front of your kids. This
is an adult decision and situation.

▼   **Be organized.** Know what the facts of your
circumstances are before you sit down.

Understand the laws that affect you by reading this book and sharing it with your partner.

▼ **Accept the limits of your situation.** There is only so much money and so much property and it has to get divided between you and your partner.

▼ **Don't beat a dead horse.** If you're not getting anywhere, stop and try again later. It will take you at least several meetings to reach decisions about all of the things in front of you. It might be helpful to set a time limit on each session so that you'll be forced to stop.

▼ **Focus on options.** Thinking of as many possible solutions as you can will give you and your partner more things to choose from, and increase the chances that you will find a solution that is mutually agreeable.

▼ **Use a list.** Create a list of things you need to work out or issues in front of you. Work your way down the list. This will keep you focused and give you a sense of accomplishment as you check things off.

Getting Help With Negotiations

There are several avenues you can take if you feel that you and your partner are not getting anywhere by negotiating on your own.

A Friend

If you have a mutual friend whom you trust, ask him or her to sit down with the both of you and help you go through the decisions. He or she can help you move through the problems and maybe point out things you aren't seeing. This may be a lot to ask of someone who loves both of you though, so be sure to only approach people you think can handle it. Having a third person in the room can help de-escalate things and force you to focus on the issues. He or she can act as a neutral party who just tries to keep the process moving forward and who makes sure you are listening to each other and understanding what the other person is saying.

❖Ron and Will were breaking up and there was a lot of hostility between them. They both agreed that they wanted to stay away from the court system, but whenever they sat down to work out an agreement, Ron would become very emotional and Will would get angry. It seemed as though there was no solution in sight until Ron happened to mention what was going on to their pastor, Jon. He was not gay, but many members of the congregation were and he was respected by all. Jon offered to sit down with Ron and Will and try to help them work out a settlement. Jon's presence changed the whole dynamic and they were able to stop focusing on emotional issues and deal with the decisions before them. It took a few meetings, but they were eventually able to decide on everything and go their separate ways.

A Mediator

A mediator is a trained professional who acts as a neutral third party and guides you and your partner though all the decisions facing you. Mediators help you generate solutions and encourage you to think creatively about your situation. Mediators usually have backgrounds in law or therapy.

They charge an hourly rate, which varies across the country, but can range from $90 to $200 an hour depending on geographic area. The goal of mediation will be a written agreement listing all of your decisions and choices. If you are legally unioned in some way, this agreement can be converted to a divorce or end of civil union agreement.

To find a mediator, you can contact the Association for Conflict Resolution (*www.acrnet.org*). Additionally, most states and major cities have mediation associations and can provide a referral in your area. When selecting a mediator, choose one who has worked with gay or lesbian couples before. See Chapter 13 for more information about mediation.

A Lawyer

If all other attempts at negotiation fail, or if you are not able to handle the paperwork needed to dissolve your legal relationship, an attorney is your best option. Expect to pay between $150 and $300 an hour for an experienced attorney's time. It is important that you find an attorney who has handled gay divorces successfully in the past. For a referral, contact your state or local bar association or ask friends if they know of anyone who specializes in gay issues. If your friends have no suggestions, try looking in your local gay phone book or check ads and sponsors in programs or other GLBT community events.

Chapter 3

Ending a Marriage

Currently the only state allowing a true legal marriage between partners of the same sex is Massachusetts. However, Canada does allow gay marriages as well, and marrying in Canada is a popular choice. When you enter into a marriage, you are required to get a formal divorce if you want to end your relationship. The problem with this, of course, is that few other states will recognize your marriage as being legal and only a few will permit you to use their divorce procedure to end your marriage. So, married couples are often left with the choice of traveling back to the place where they got married, or simply separating without legally ending their marriage. It can be difficult to know what you can do and how to make a choice. The best way is to learn about the divorce processes in the places where marriages are permitted and decide if this is a process you want or are able to take part in.

Massachusetts

Should you end your Massachusetts marriage? If your relationship has ended and you were married in Massachusetts, you are probably trying to decide if you need to get a divorce or not. If you live in Massachusetts or possibly Vermont, or if it would be relatively easy for you to establish residency in either of these two states, you should seriously consider getting a divorce or dissolution in one of these states. If you are a resident of Massachusetts, you can't file your state taxes as a single person unless you get a divorce. Also, your spouse still has the right to inherit from your estate unless you divorce. However if you live in another state where your marriage is not recognized, you cannot obtain a divorce there (although there are many, many test cases working their way through the courts right now and this may change any day). The Connecticut Attorney General has issused an opinion that the state will not recognize Massachusettes marriages so, at this point, you would not be able to get a divorce in Connecticut.

Legal Process and Paperwork

In Massachusetts you can end your marriage by divorce or annulment.

Annulment

To obtain an annulment, or a legal decision that your marriage was never valid in the first place, you must prove that:

▼ You are related to each other in a way that would preclude marriage.

▼ One of you was underage at the time of the marriage.

▼ One of you was suffering from insanity or idiocy at the time of the marriage.

▼ The marriage was begun under fraud or duress, or involved impotency, concealment of a pregnancy, or concealment of contagious diseases.

Residency and Jurisdiction

To be able to get a Massachusetts divorce, you must satisfy the residency requirements. To qualify, you must be able to prove that:

▼ You lived in Massachusetts as a spouse.

▼ The cause of action for your divorce arose in Massachusetts (meaning the reasons for the divorce happened in the state).

▼ One spouse lives in the state and the cause of action arose in the state.

▼ The person filing for divorce has lived in the state for one year prior to filing.

Massachusetts divorce cases must be filed in the state probate and family courts. To locate a courthouse, see: *www.mass.gov/courts/courtsandjudges/courts/ probateandfamilycourt/courtcounty.html*.

To begin the case, a complaint is filed. At the time of the filing, you do not need to be living apart from each other.

Grounds

The reasons, or grounds, that can be used legally in Massachusetts for divorce are the following:

▼ Irretrievable breakdown of the marriage (this is the no-fault provision).

▼ Cruel and inhuman treatment.

▼ Nonsupport (this is a failure to financially support the other spouse).

▼ Desertion for one year, adultery, impotency, addiction, or imprisonment for five years or more.

Most couples choose the irretrievable breakdown reason because you do not need to assign blame. If you use this provision, you can proceed in two ways:

▼ File a no-fault petition signed by both of you and your attorney and a sworn affidavit with a notarized separation agreement. Then have a court hearing to review the documents. A decision is issued within 30 days of the hearing and the divorce is final.

▼ File a petition without a separation agreement (if you haven't been able to come to an agreement) and have a trial within six months after the initial filing.

There is a $215 fee to file a complaint for divorce, in addition to other fees throughout the process. If you cannot afford these fees, Massachusetts has a process for declaring a person indigent so that all court fees are waived.

To file papers in Massachusetts you must be able to provide the following information:

▼ Names.

▼ Current addresses.

▼ Dates of birth.

▼ Date of marriage.

▼ Social Security numbers.

▼ Names and dates of birth of children born into the marriage or in the custody of either spouse.

Forms for divorce are available online at: *www.lawlib.state.ma.us/forms.html#divorce*. Also try *www.hampshireprobate.com/Divorce%20Info/ uncontested_divorce.htm*. A checklist of no-fault forms is available at: *www.lawlib.state.ma.us/divorce.html*.

Child Support

You can find the Massachusetts child support guidelines online at: *www.mass.gov/courts/formsandguidelines/ csg2002.html.*

The basic obligation in Massachusetts is 21 percent of income if there is one child, 24 percent if there are two children and, 27 percent if there are three or more children. This amount is calculated based on the noncustodial parent's income, but is then adjusted by considering the custodial parent's income. The amount of child support increases as the child ages.

Custody

Massachusetts uses a best interests analysis to determine custody. Custody in Massachusetts is divided in the following ways:

▼ **Sole legal custody:** One parent has the right and responsibility to make major decisions such as the child's education, medical care, and emotional, moral, and religious development.

▼ **Shared legal custody:** There is continued mutual responsibility and involvement by both parents in major decisions about the child's welfare including education, medical care, and emotional, moral, and religious development.

▼ **Sole physical custody:** The child lives with one parent, and has reasonable visitation with the other parent, unless the court determines that such visitation would not be in the best interest of the child.

▼ **Shared physical custody:** The child spends time with both and there is frequent and continued contact with both parents. Normally the child has primary residence at the home of one of the parents.

When deciding custody, the court must consider whether anyone in the family abuses alcohol or drugs or has ever deserted the child. The court also considers if the spouses have a history of being able and willing to cooperate about things involving the child. The happiness and welfare of the child is another important consideration and the court looks at whether the child's present or past living conditions adversely affect his physical, mental, moral, or emotional health. Children more than 14 years of age are permitted to have a voice in the custody proceeding.

Massachusetts requires all parents involved in custody cases to attend Parent Education Programs. These classes are designed to help parents understand the effect of divorce on children and encourage them to work together as parents even after the divorce. A list of approved programs can be found at: *www.mass.gov/courts/courtsandjudges/courts/ probateandfamilycourt/parented.html*.

Property Division

Both parties must complete a financial statement. The short form can be used if your income is under $75,000. Information on filling out this form is available at: *www.neighborhoodlaw.org/page/58043&cat_id=35*. Massachusetts is an equitable distribution state which means marital property is divided in a way that is fair, but not necessarily 50/50. The factors that are considered by a court in dividing property are the same as those used in deciding alimony which will be discussed later in this chapter.

Massachusetts also has a statute that allows the court to order one spouse to vacate the marital home for 90 days initially if the health, safety, or welfare of the person asking, or any children, would be in danger without the order. The person being asked to leave has to be given three days notice of the hearing.

Alimony

Massachusetts will grant alimony payments or a lump sum. Massachusetts courts can award alimony at the time of the divorce. When considering alimony, the court must take into consideration:

▼ The length of the marriage.

▼ The conduct of the parties during the marriage.

▼ The age of the parties.

▼ The health of the parties.

▼ The station, occupation, amount and sources of income, vocational skills, employability, estate, liabilities, and needs of each of the parties and the opportunity of each for future acquisition of capital assets and income.

▼ The present and future needs of the dependent children of the marriage.

▼ The contribution of each of the parties in the acquisition, preservation, or appreciation in value of their respective estates and the contribution of each of the parties as a home-maker to the family unit.

The court can also order one spouse to pay for health insurance for the other spouse, if it is available at a reasonable cost. The court can order the spouse with health insurance to use the option of a family plan or reimburse the noninsured spouse for the cost of buying health insurance.

Finding Legal Assistance

To find an attorney, contact the Massachusetts Bar Association Lawyer Referral Service at (800) 392-6164. The service allows you to set up a 30 minute consultation with an attorney for $25. Free help is also available on the first Wednesday of each month, from 5:30 to 7:30 p.m., when volunteer lawyers are available to answer basic legal questions by phone. Dial-a-Lawyer may be reached at (617) 338-0610.

Representing Yourself

If you choose to represent yourself in Massachusetts, ask for assistance from the court personnel in filing forms. Massachusetts courthouses can be located online at: *www.mass.gov/courts/courtsandjudges/courts/ probateandfamilycourt/courtcounty.html*.

Mediation

Mediation is an excellent way to create a separation agreement that can be filed with the court in a no-fault divorce. To find a mediator, go to: *www.mass.gov/courts/ courtsandjudges/courts/probateandfamilycourt/ adrlisting.html*.

Legal Effect

If you divorce in Massachusetts, the terms of the divorce may be honored by states such as Vermont, as well as some other states that have not formally recognized same sex marriage and divorce.

Canada

If you were married in Canada, you can get a divorce in Canada. You must live in Canada for one year before you are eligible to file for divorce. You can, however, file in Massachusetts or Vermont, because these states will most likely recognize a Canadian same sex marriage. Divorce laws in Canada are governed by the federal Divorce Act and each province then has its own procedures and regulations. If you were married in one province, you can divorce in another province after meeting the one year residency requirement. At the time this book was written, same sex marriage had just been legalized throughout Canada, so in many provinces there have not yet been any same sex divorces.

Annulment

Canada permits annulments when there was mistaken or false representation about a person's identity, status, or habits. Absence of consent, incompetence, mistake, and consanguinity (being related) may all be grounds for annulment. Each province also has specific laws about annulment, so if this is something you are interested in, you need to talk to an attorney in the province in which you will be seeking the annulment.

Residency and Jurisdiction

Canadian courts have jurisdiction over a divorce case if one of the parties has lived in that province for at least one year before filing. In British Columbia, the Yukon and Northwest Territories, the Supreme Court [Trial Division] has the power to hear divorces. In Ontario, this court is called the Ontario Court [General Division] and in Quebec, it is called the Superior Court.

Grounds

There is one ground for divorce in Canada: breakdown of the marriage. There are three different subcategories of this however:

▼ The spouses have lived apart for at least one year immediately preceding the divorce judgment (this is the no-fault provision).

▼ The defendant spouse has committed adultery.

▼ One spouse has treated the other with physical or mental cruelty that has made continuation of the marriage intolerable.

At any point in the process you can live together again for up to 90 days for the purpose of reconciliation and if it doesn't work out, it does not affect your proceeding.

Property Division

In Canada marital property is supposed to be distributed in an equal way.

Custody

Custody in Canada is determined based on the best interests of the children. The court takes into consideration the condition, means, needs, and other circumstances of the child. Courts try to grant maximum contact with both parents whenever possible. The court usually leans toward giving custody to a parent who can provide full-time care rather than a parent who will put the child in day care.

Child Support

Guidelines for child and spousal support can be found online at *canada.justice.gc.ca/en/ps/sup/grl/ligfed.html*. Forms and information about child and spousal support can be found at *www.ccra-adrc.ca*.

Citizenship

If you became a Canadian citizen after marrying a Canadian, getting a divorce will not change your citizenship.

Legal Help

To find a Canadian lawyer, contact the Canadian Bar Lawyer Referral at: *www.cba.org/BC/Initiatives/main/lawyer_Referral.aspx*. A pamphlet on Canadian divorce is available at *www.canada.justice.gc.ca/en/dept/pub/divorce/DOJ.pdf*.

Province Specific Forms and Legal Assistance

Alberta

The Court of Queen's Bench hears divorce cases. If you would like to find forms pertaining to divorce or other legal matters, they can be found online at *www.albertacourts.ab.ca.go.aspx?tabid=350*. Legal assistance and information is also available at *www.albertacourts.ab.ca/familylaw/* or (780) 415-0404. Mediation services are available at *www.albertacourts.ab.ca/go.aspx?tabid=544* or (403) 297-698.

British Columbia

Forms can be found at *www.familylaw.lss.bc.ca/selfhelpmaterials.asp*.

Legal Services BC is available online at *www.lss.bc.ca/* or you can call Lawline at (604) 408-2172 (Lower Mainland) (866) 577-2525 (toll free, outside the Lower Mainland). After your call connects, press "7" to reach to LawLINE.

Manitoba

Forms can be found online at *http://web2.gov.mb.ca/laws/rules/70ae.html* and information about Manitoba divorce courts can be found at *www.manitobacourts.mb.ca/english/faq/faq_family_div.html*. For legal assistance in Manitoba, contact Legal Aid at *www.legalaid.mb.ca/* or (800) 261-2960. Legal Referral can be contacted at *www.communitylegal.mb.ca/refer.asp* or (800) 262-8800.

Ontario

Forms for Ontario divorces can be found online at: *www.ontariocourts.on.ca/family_court/forms/*. The Ontario Lawyer Referral Program can be reached at *www.lsuc.on.ca/public/a/finding/* or by calling (900) 565-4LRS (4577).

New Brunswick

A list of area legal aid offices is available online at *www.gnb.ca/cour/domestic-e.asp*. A list of mediation services is available at *www.gnb.ca/cour/04CQB/Mediation-e.asp*. The lawyer referral program can be accessed at *www.lawsociety.nb.ca/* or (506) 458-8540. Forms are available online at *www.gnb.ca/0062/regs/Form/form_liste.htm*.

Newfoundland and Labrador

Forms can be found online at *www.justice.gov.nl.ca/ just/CIVIL/family_law.htm*.

For legal assistance, contact Legal Aid at *www.justice.gov.nl.ca/just/Other/otherx/legalaid.htm* or (800) 563-9911.

Or you can contact Lawyer Referral at *www.publiclegalinfo.com/services.html* or (709) 722-2643.

Nova Scotia

Forms are located online at *www.courts.ns.ca/self_rep/ self_rep_kits.htm*.

Lawyer Referral is available at *www.legalinfo.org/ referral.html* or (800) 665-9779.

Prince Edward Island

Cases are heard in the Supreme Court, Trial Division. Forms are available online at *www.gov.pe.ca/courts/ supreme/index.php3?number=1003815*. A lawyer referral service is available at *www.isn.net/cliapei/79.html* or (800) 240-9798.

Quebec

Forms for Quebec divorce can be found online at: *www.justice.gouv.qc.ca/english/publications/generale/dem-conj-mod-a.htm*. Legal assistance is available only in French at: *www.barreau.qc.ca/infos/default.asp*.

Saskatchewan

The self-help divorce kit and forms are available for a fee at local Court of the Queen's Bench Registrar's Offices.

They are not available online. Look in the government section of the phone book to locate a court near you.

Legal aid is available at *www.legalaid.sk.ca/* and lawyer referral is available at *www.lawsociety.sk.ca/NewLook/Programs/referral.htm.* or (800) 667-9886.

Yukon Territory

A self-help kit and forms are available in person or by mail for a $5 fee at:

Supreme Court Court Registry Law Courts, 2134 Second Avenue (ground floor), Whitehorse, Yukon Y1A 5H6. Phone: (867) 667-5937; Toll-free within Yukon, (800) 661-0408, ext. 5937. E-mail: courtservices@gov.yk.ca

For legal help contact the Law Society of Yukon. Phone: (867) 668-4231 or find the lawyer referral online at *www.lawsocietyyukon.com/referral.asp*.

Chapter 4

Ending a Civil Union

At the time this book was written, two states had made civil unions legal: Vermont and Connecticut. To end a civil union, you must follow that state's divorce process.

Should You End Your Union?

Before you go through the time and expense of divorcing, you should carefully consider whether it is worthwhile for you to do so. If you are a Vermont or Connecticut resident, ending your civil union does make sense, because if you do not, you are still legally joined in the eyes of your state. You must file joint state taxes, continue to have inheritance rights from each other, and are required to support each other.

If you are not a resident, your union has no effect in the state you are living in (unless you're in Massachusetts, which recognizes civil unions). The fact that you have a civil union has no impact on your rights within your own state (because it doesn't recognize same sex marriage), so ending the union will also have no impact on your rights in your own state. Your union isn't going to be upheld in your state and it has no legal meaning there.

While this is the legal perspective, you need to look at it from a personal perspective as well. Many couples feel bound to each other unless they dissolve the union. The simple fact that you took those vows probably means something to you and you might not feel able to go on with your separate lives unless you take formal steps to dissolve the union. Should you meet someone new and eventually decide you want to marry or get a civil union again, you will need to dissolve this union first to be able to enter into that one.

In Salucco v. Alldredge, a Massachusetts court dissolved a Vermont civil union. If you live in Massachusetts or establishing residence there would be easier for you, you may wish to read the chapter about Massachusetts divorce and consider dissolving your union there under Massachusetts law. Gay and Lesbian Advocates and Defenders (GLAD) believes that Rhode Island will recognize same sex unions from other states, but this has not yet been tested. Texas courts have refused to dissolve civil unions, but West Virginia granted a civil union divorce in 2002.

Because this is a constantly evolving area of law, it is very possible that other states will dissolve civil unions granted elsewhere, but the only way to know for sure is for test cases to go forward. Many states have cases that are in the legal process right now, and many states have laws for gay divorce and civil unions still pending at this current time.

❖Merc and Randy live in Missouri and went to Vermont to get a civil union. Within a year though, their partnership had ended. Randy had found someone else and had moved out. Their split was not amicable and they haven't spoken since. Merc looked into getting a Vermont divorce, but there was just no way he could leave his job and move there for a year. He felt he had no other options, so decided to leave it be for now. Because their state does not recognize their union, getting a dissolution offers them no benefits right now. Merc does think that if he ever falls in love again and wants to get married that he may feel it's necessary to get the Vermont union dissolved, but hopes that by then there will be some more affordable options available to him.

It is possible to seek a divorce in your home state, but as Kimberly Jean Brown and Jennifer Sue Perez of Iowa have discovered, it will be controversial and may not be upheld. Brown and Perez got a civil union in Vermont and returned to their home state of Iowa. They decided to separate and sought a divorce in the Iowa District Court. Judge Neary signed the divorce order saying that under the full faith and credit act of the Constitution, Iowa must recognize marriages in other states and grant divorces for them. At the time this book was written however, an appeal by Iowa state lawmakers was pending. The lawmakers allege that because Iowa has a defense of marriage act, same sex unions are not recognized and cannot be granted Iowa divorces. The appeal is still pending and Lambda Legal has filed a brief asking the court to uphold the divorce ruling. The only certain way to dissolve a Vermont civil union at this point is by obtaining a Vermont divorce. Test cases are needed in every state to press this issue and create awareness and case law that will make divorce widely available to all gay couples.

Vermont

Residency

To get a divorce in Vermont you must meet the state residency requirement. One of you must have lived in Vermont for at least six months at the time of filing and at least 12 months at the time the divorce is finalized. This requirement is your biggest barrier if you are from out of state. One of you is going to have to move to Vermont for at least one year. This can be quite a burden, but there is no way around it. If your partner files for divorce in Vermont, he or she is the one who must meet the residency requirement, not you. If you're served with papers for a Vermont divorce, you will have to appear in court there for the divorce, but you don't have to meet any residency requirement.

Grounds

There are several choices when it comes to the reason you give the court for divorce in Vermont. Vermont has a no-fault option, which means neither of you is considered to have caused the union to end. This option is available only if you have lived apart for six months before filing. A no-fault divorce can help avoid a lot of unpleasantness because no one has to say anything bad about the other person.

There are a variety of options for a fault divorce, including: adultery, imprisonment for three years or more or for life, willful desertion for seven years, cruel and inhuman treatment of intolerable severity, incurable mental illness, and gross neglect. When you choose a fault divorce, you will be required to give testimony about the reason and cite specific instances.

Read Vermont divorce and annulment statutes online at *www.leg.state.vt.us/statutes/chapters.cfm?Title=15.*

Paperwork

On average, it takes about 15 months for a Vermont divorce to proceed through the necessary legal channels. The process beings when you or your partner files a summons or complaint with the court in the county where either of you resides (remember you have to be a Vermont resident to file). The other partner is then notified that the divorce has been filed. This is done by formal service of process in which a process server will usually physically hand him or her the papers. It is still possible to get a divorce if you can't find or have your partner served. Other methods include a court order to publish the summons instead of serving it, but if you are having trouble serving or locating your partner, you need to speak to a Vermont attorney to review your options.

To file for divorce, you need to know both spouse's birth dates, the date and place of the union, the legal residence of both parties, and select a reason for the divorce. If you are the partner who filed, you will be required to complete a complaint, which is a document explaining why you are ending the union and what issues you are asking the court to decide (such as property division or custody).

Once papers have been filed and the other party has been served, pretrial orders are filed with the court. These are temporary orders that allow the judge to make a temporary decision about things such as custody and visitation, or financial support. These orders will stay in place until the final decision is reached in the case. The next step in the process is the discovery phase when your attorney will gather evidence and information that will explain to the court why you should get what you are asking for. Once information is gathered, your attorney will most likely try to reach a settlement with your partner's attorney. Doing so will not only save you money, but will also avoid the emotional stress and the added cost of a trial.

If you will be having a trial, you will first have a pretrial hearing where the judge or a group of attorneys will try to help you reach a settlement. If that isn't successful then you will have a trial in front of a judge (not a jury). Each side will have a turn to present witnesses and evidence and you will need to testify. The judge will then make his or her decision, indicate how all of the issues are decided, and your civil union will be formally ended.

You have the right to appeal the decision in your case if you don't agree with it and it is important that you discuss this with your attorney because there are rigid time restrictions on appeals.

Annulment

Annulment is another option available in Vermont. The civil union annulment process is the same as it is for straight couples.

You can annul your civil union if:

▼ One of you was underage at the time the union was created.

▼ One of you is an idiot or a lunatic (these really are the words used in the law!).

▼ One of you was physically incapable of entering into the union.

▼ Fraud or force was used to get one of the parties to consent to the union.

These requirements are ways of showing that you both didn't enter into the union willingly and knowingly. Because of this, the union was never valid or real.

To obtain an annulment, you must be a resident of the state of Vermont (and have lived there at least six months— there's that burdensome requirement again). You will need to hire an attorney who can file the annulment papers for you and you may need to provide medical records to prove lunacy or physical incapacity. Annulments usually occur soon after a union, so there is rarely a need to divide joint property because there isn't much time to acquire it. If you have children together and you are both legal parents, the children are considered legal children of the union (in other words, they are not illegitimate) and a custody decision, as well as a child support decision, can be made by the court.

Your Rights in a Vermont Divorce

Vermont treats a civil union divorce exactly the same as a straight divorce, so you will be governed by all the state laws that apply to divorce. You won't be treated any differently or held to different standards. Between 2000 and 2002 there were only 13 civil union divorces in Vermont, so it is still a relatively rare occurrence. But just because it's rare doesn't mean it's not available.

Property Division

Vermont is an "equitable distribution" state, meaning that all property acquired during the union must be divided in a way that is fair, if not necessarily equal. You're not automatically entitled to half, but you are entitled to an amount that is fair in your circumstances. When dividing property, the court will consider:

▼ The contribution of each spouse to the acquisition of the property, including the contribution of each spouse as homemaker.

▼ The value of each spouse's property.

▼ The length of the union.

▼ The age and health of the spouses.

▼ The occupation of the spouses.

▼ The amount and sources of income of the spouses.

▼ The vocational skills of the spouses.

▼ The employability of the spouses.

▼ The liabilities and needs of each spouse and the opportunity of each for further acquisition of capital assets and income.

▼ Whether the property award is instead of, or in addition to, maintenance.

▼ How and by whom the property was acquired.

▼ The merits of each spouse.

▼ Any custodial provisions for the children, including the desirability of awarding the family home to the parent with custody of any children.

▼ The contribution by one spouse to the education, training, or increased earning power of the other.

Chapter 9 will help you work through property division issues.

Spousal Support

Spousal support is not as common as it used to be, but you are entitled to ask for it. Generally it's only ordered when one spouse needs help becoming financially stable after the union ends. The court will only order it if the spouse seeking it: (1) lacks sufficient income or property to provide for his or her reasonable needs and (2) is unable to support him or herself through appropriate employment at the standard of living established during the union or is the custodian of any children.

The court will consider the following factors in deciding the amount of spousal support:

▼ The time necessary to acquire sufficient education and training to enable the spouse to find appropriate employment, and that spouse's future earning capacity.

▼ The standard of living established during the union.

▼ The duration of the union.

▼ The ability of the spouse from whom support is sought to meet his or her needs while meeting those of the spouse seeking support.

▼ The financial resources of the spouse seeking maintenance, including property apportioned to the spouse and the spouse's ability to meet his or her needs independently.

▼ The age of the spouses.

▼ The physical and emotional conditions of the spouses.

▼ The effects of inflation on the cost of living.

See Chapter 12 for a complete discussion about spousal support.

Custody

If custody and visitation is an issue in your case, joint or sole child custody may be awarded based on the best interests of the child, and the consideration by the court of all relevant factors, including the following:

▼ The wishes of the parents.

▼ The child's adjustment to his or her home, school, and community.

▼ The relationship of the child with parents, siblings, and other significant family members.

▼ The ability and disposition of each parent to provide love, affection, and guidance.

▼ The ability of each parent to provide food, clothing, medical care, other material needs, and a safe environment.

▼ The ability of each parent to meet the child's present and future developmental needs.

▼ The ability and disposition of each parent to foster a positive relationship and frequent and continuing contact with the other parent, including physical contact unless, it will result in harm to the child or parent.

▼ The quality of the child's relationship with the primary care provider, given the child's age and development.

▼ The ability and disposition of the parents to communicate, cooperate with each other, and make joint decisions concerning the children where parental rights and responsibilities are to be shared.

Under Vermont law neither parent is assumed to have a superior right to have custody and courts do not favor stay at home parents over working parents. See Chapter 10 for more information about custody and how divorce affects your child.

Child Support

If child support is an issue in your case, either or both of you may be required to pay child support. The court considers the following factors when deciding child support:

▼ The financial resources of the child.

▼ The standard of living the child would have enjoyed if the union had not been dissolved.

▼ The physical and emotional conditions and educational needs of the child.

▼ The financial resources, needs, and obligations of both the noncustodial and the custodial parent.

▼ Inflation with relation to the cost of living.

▼ The costs of any educational needs of either parent.

▼ Any travel expenses related to parent-child contact.

The court can order that health insurance coverage be provided for the child. The court can also require that child support be paid by wage deduction. Child support amounts are based on income guidelines set up by the state and increase with the number of children you have. Read the current guidelines online at *www.ocs.state.vt.us.* More information about how child support is calculated and how to negotiate it is provided in Chapter 11.

Finding Legal Assistance

If you plan to seek a divorce in Vermont, you will need an attorney who is licensed to practice in Vermont. If you live in Vermont, get referrals from friends and family. If you're from out of state and have few connections in Vermont, contact: The Vermont Bar Association, 35-37 Court Street, P.O. Box 100, Montpelier, VT 05601-0100. Or go online to *www.vtbar.org*. The Lawyer Referral Program can be reached at (800) 639-7036, or e-mail nredington@vtbar.org

The referral program will refer you to an attorney who is experienced in this area of law.

Representing Yourself

It is possible to represent yourself in a Vermont divorce. Vermont is very supportive of people who wish to represent themselves in court. Vermont Family Court offers a pro se education class (pro se is a Latin term that just means you're representing yourself), that is designed to help you understand the ins and outs of handling your case yourself. The class is held in different counties on different days, so you will need to contact your local family court (see later in this chapter for contact information) to find out when the next class in your area is. You can obtain the forms you need for your case online at *www.vermontjudiciary.org/eforms/default.aspx* or at your local family court. Free online assistance is available at *www.vtlawhelp.org*.

Using Mediation

Mediation is an alternative to a contested divorce. A mediator helps you and your partner reach agreements about all of the issues involved in your divorce. These agreements are then approved by the court and your union is dissolved. You avoid contested court proceedings and also save money on attorney fees. Vermont also has a Family

Mediation Project, which makes trained mediators available to those involved in divorces. Find out more about the program at *www.vermontjudiciary.org/mediation/* or by calling (800) 622-6359. More information about using mediation to end your union is in Chapter 13.

❖Colette and Jenn are Vermont residents who got a civil union. When their relationship ended, they got a dissolution. Both were surprised at how smoothly it went for them. They both had lawyers who explained that their case would be handled like any other Vermont divorce. The court divided their property, arranged custody of their children, and ordered child support. Even though the court procedure worked very smoothly, the process was an emotionally difficult one for both of them.

Connecticut

The Connecticut civil union law grants the same rights to same sex civil union couples as heterosexual married couples, thus the procedures for a civil union dissolution will be the same as those for a marriage in Connecticut.

Residency

Connecticut has a residency requirement for divorce, which apply to civil unions: one spouse must be a resident for one year, one spouse was a resident at the time of the civil union and returned with the intention of having a permanent residence there, or the grounds for the dissolution arose in Connecticut.

Grounds

The grounds for divorce or dissolution in Connecticut are:

▼ Irretrievable breakdown of the marriage (this is a no-fault provision).

▼ Incompatibility and voluntary separation for 18 months with no reasonable prospect for reconciliation (another no-fault provision).

▼ Adultery.

▼ Life imprisonment or commission and/or conviction of an infamous crime involving a violation of conjugal duty and imprisonment for at least one year.

▼ Hospitalization or institutionalization for mental illness for a total of five years.

▼ Willful desertion and nonsupport for one year.

▼ Seven years absence.

▼ Intolerable cruelty.

▼ Fraud.

▼ Habitual intemperance (alcohol addiction).

Divorces and civil union dissolutions are handled by the Superior Court of Connecticut. To use the no-fault option, you must both sign a statement that the marriage is irretrievably broken, and file it with the court. If requested, the court will order the case to go to mediation.

Annulment

Annulment is available if the marriage was void under state requirements: one party was under the age of 18; the parties are related to each other and fraud or duress was used to compel one person to agree to the marriage.

Separation

In Connecticut, you can seek a legal separation instead of a divorce if you wish. The process is exactly the same, except that your decree declares you legally separated, not divorced. You still must file state taxes as a married person. Also, you still have the right to inherit from each other but the court will decide all issues of support, custody, and property division.

Your Rights in a Connecticut Divorce

Property Distribution

Connecticut uses an equitable distribution theory and decides how to distribute property based on the following factors:

▼ The contribution of each spouse to the acquisition of the marital property, including the contribution of each spouse as homemaker.

▼ The length of the marriage.

▼ The age and health of the spouses.

▼ The occupation of the spouses.

▼ The amount and sources of income of the spouses.

▼ The vocational skills of the spouses.

▼ The employability of the spouses.

▼ The estate, liabilities, and needs of each spouse and the opportunity of each for further acquisition of capital assets and income.

▼ The circumstances that contributed to the estrangement of the spouses.

▼ The causes of the dissolution of marriage.

▼ The contribution of each of the parties in acquiring or preserving assets.

Alimony

When considering whether to order alimony, the court must consider the following factors:

▼ The length of the marriage.

▼ The causes for the annulment, dissolution of the marriage, or legal separation.

▼ The age, health, station, occupation, amount and sources of income, vocational skills, employability, estate, and needs of each of the parties.

▼ The property distribution.

In the case of a parent to whom the custody of minor children has been awarded, the desirability of the parent's securing employment would be considered as a major factor (if the court feels it makes sense for a parent to stay at home with a child, an award would be higher).

Custody

The court can consider the wishes of the child if he or she is old enough and may also consider the reasons for the divorce if it has an impact on the child. Beyond this, there are no required considerations and the judge must use the best interests analysis. (See Chapter 10 for more information about the best interests analysis.)

Child Support

The following factors must be considered when deciding child support:

▼ The financial resources of the child.

▼ The age, health, and station of the parents.

▼ The occupation of each parent.

▼ The earning capacity of each parent.

▼ The amount and sources of income of each parent.

▼ The vocational skills and employability of each parent.

▼ The age and health of the child.

▼ The child's occupation.

▼ The vocational skills of the child.

▼ The employability of the child.

▼ The estate and needs of the child.

▼ The relative financial means of the parents.

Paperwork

A divorce case begins by filing a complaint, which must be served on the other party. There is a 90 day waiting period from the date the complaint is filed until the case can actually be heard. Spouses can ask the judge to order that they both participate in a reconciliation conference, to try and save the marriage. Superior Court hears divorce cases in Connecticut. You can find Superior Court forms online at: *http://jud2.state.ct.us/webforms/#family*. Addresses and contact information are available at: *www.jud.state.ct.us/external/super/default.htm*.

Getting Help

You can get a referral to a Connecticut attorney online through the Connecticut Bar Association Lawyer Referral Program at *www.ctbar.org/article/articleview/291*. To read an overview of the divorce process, see *www.ctbar.org/article/articleview/247.* Connecticut has Court Service Centers that are set up to help people who will be representing themselves in court. To find one, see *www.jud.state.ct.us/directory/directory/servcenter.htm* or call (860) 563-9435, ext. 359. You can find out more about Connecticut divorce laws online at *www.cga.ct.gov/2005/ pubChap815j.htm#Sec46b-40.htm.*

Connecticut has a court mediation program and you can request that your case be referred to it. For more information, see *www.jud.state.ct.us/external/super/ altdisp.htm* or call (860) 563-9435, ext. 315.

Chapter 5
Ending a Registered Domestic Partnership

There are many different kinds of domestic partnerships across the United States. This chapter examines the state programs. If you registered your domestic partnership with a municipality, contact the town or city clerk for information on how to dissolve it. In most cases, filing a simple form will be all you need to do.

Maine Domestic Partnerships

If you registered your domestic partnership in Maine, and live in Maine, you need to file for a termination because the law gives you rights to each other's estate. If you do not live in Maine, there may be no reason for you to terminate. There are several ways you can terminate your partnership in Maine.

Termination by Marriage

If either of you enter into a marriage (the law does not specify that this must be a heterosexual marriage, but most likely this is how it will be interpreted because

Maine does not recognize same sex marriages), your domestic partnership is terminated.

Termination With Consent

If you both agree you want to terminate your partnership, you must complete the Termination of Domestic Partnership by Mutual Consent Form and sign it in front of a notary. This form is then filed with the Office of Vital Records, along with a $35 fee.

Termination Without Consent

If you have been unable to agree to terminate your partnership or have been unable to agree about the details of your termination, you can use what is called Alternate Notice of Termination of Domestic Partnership. To use this method, you serve (either hand it to your partner, or use one of the methods of legal service, such as using a process server) your partner a photocopy of the form. File the original along with the proof of service form. Wait 60 days and your termination is effective.

If you don't give notice, you can be held liable for any monetary losses your partner incurs, such as late fees on bills or rent that result from the failure to give notice.

Getting Help

Forms and filing instructions are available online at: *www.maine.gov/dhhs/bohodr/domstcprtnrspge.htm*.

❖ Katrina and Lil had a Maine domestic partnership. Lil packed up and moved out overnight. Katrina was in shock for weeks. Although she realized it was unlikely Lil was coming back,
continued on next page

she still held onto a shred of hope. One day she was legally served with a notice that Lil was filing for a dissolution. Katrina did not want a dissolution and instead hoped they could find a way to work out their problems. She went to see a lawyer to ask what she could do to stop the dissolution. Basically he told her she had little chance of being able to stop it. She could file a case seeking a temporary order halting the dissolution and then try to convince the court that it should not be granted, but because Maine law does not require consent, only notice, it was almost certain she would lose. Katrina did nothing and her partnership was dissolved.

New Jersey Domestic Partnerships

New Jersey recognizes civil unions and domestic partnerships from other states if the partners live together and provide support for each other, are jointly responsible for living expenses, neither is married, they are not related, they are the same sex, they are 18 or older, they file an Affidavit of Domestic Partnership, and neither has been in a partnership that ended within the last 180 days. If your partnership is recognized by New Jersey, you can file for termination in New Jersey.

If you registered your domestic partnership in New Jersey and you live in New Jersey, you need to terminate it because the law makes you responsible for each other's support as long as you are partners. If you do not live in New Jersey, there may be no reason to terminate. You cannot register with another partner for 180 days after dissolving a partnership in New Jersey.

To obtain a New Jersey dissolution, you must have grounds, or a reason. The reasons permitted are the same as those used for marriage:

▼ **Voluntary separation for 18 months.** This is the no-fault provision and allows you to dissolve your partnership once you have lived apart in separate houses for 18 months and have no hope of reconciliation.

▼ **Extreme Cruelty.** Mental or physical cruelty which makes it unreasonable or improper for you to continue to live together.

▼ **Adultery.** One of the partners had voluntary sexual intercourse with someone else.

▼ **Desertion.** One partner has deserted the other for at least 12 months and they have stopped living as partners.

▼ **Addiction.** Controlled substances or alcohol qualify and the addiction must have been going on for 12 months.

▼ **Institutionalization.** One spouse is hospitalized for mental illness for 12 months during the partnership.

▼ **Imprisonment.** One spouse is imprisoned for at least 18 months and the partners have not resumed cohabitation.

▼ **Deviant Sexual Conduct.** One partner engages in what is called "deviant sexual conduct" without the consent of the other partner.

▼ **Age.** When both partners are more than 62 years of age and one enters into a heterosexual marriage.

To file, you must fill out a Termination of Domestic Partnership Complaint in Superior Court. The court does not have the authority to award support, or decide custody and visitation issues within this proceeding. The court has the authority to distribute property, but is not required to. This means that if you want, you can decide on a property settlement without supervision by the court, or you can ask the court to decide property division if you can't on your own. The partners have the authority to enter into a written agreement outside the terms of the statute, so you can agree to support or distribution in this agreement. You have the right to continue your health insurance if it is through your partner, using COBRA.

Your Termination of Domestic Partnership Complaint to the court must include:

▼ A statement of essential facts (that you are seeking termination and the grounds you are using).

▼ The address of each party or a statement that a current address is not known.

▼ A statement of essential facts to establish jurisdiction and venue.

▼ A statement of any previous court actions between the parties.

▼ An affidavit of insurance pursuant to R.5:4-2(f). (A listing of all insurance coverages can be found atwww.abcdivorces.com.)

▼ The date and place where the domestic partnership or other civil union was granted or registered.

▼ A request to terminate the domestic partnership.

▼ A statement of whether joint property needs to be divided.

The filing fee is currently $250. At the present time, New Jersey does not have any standard forms a pro se litigant (someone representing themselves) can use. You will need to hire an attorney to prepare a complaint and file it for you.

Domestic partners are not liable for each other's debts under the law, even debts incurred during the partnership, though partners are responsible for each other's basic needs. So when a domestic partnership ends, one partner cannot be held responsible for the other's debts. However, this is an untested area of law—if one partner ended up with debt due to medical care during the relationship this may be considered a basic need and therefore the other partner might be held responsible.

The New Jersey law does not make post-dissolution spousal support something that is required. The law makes equitable distribution of partnership property something that a judge can order, but is not required.

Getting Help

New Jersey has a court-referred mediation program. For more information on how this program can assist you, go online at *www.judiciary.state.nj.us/services/cdr.htm*. Or for guidance you can contact: Thomas N. Farrell Manager,CDR Programs Special Programs Unit, Administrative Office of the Courts, P.O.Box 988, Trenton, NJ, 08625, Telephone: (609) 984-5032. You can contact the lawyer referral program at: *www.njsba.com/lawyer_referral/*.

Hawaii Reciprocal Beneficiary Relationships

If you registered a reciprocal beneficiary relationship in Hawaii and live in Hawaii, it is a good idea to terminate your relationship because the law gives you inheritance rights when you are in a legal relationship such as this. If you live in another state, it may not make sense for you to terminate.

To end your relationship you must file a form with the state. Download the form at *www.hawaii.gov/health/ vital-records/vital-records/reciprocalindex.html*. Both of you must complete the form and have it notarized. You must file the form with the Department of Health, along with an $8 filing fee (money order or cashier's check only, made payable to the State Director of Finance, no cash or personal checks accepted). Enclose one stamped, self-addressed legal size envelope (two if you would each like separate copies at your separate addresses). Mail all of this to: RBR Office, P.O. Box 591 Honolulu, HI 96809-0591.

You cannot personally take the form in; it must be mailed (although you can stop in and personally pick up blank forms).

Two copies will be mailed in the envelope you provide. (Or one in each envelope if you enclose two.) If you need additional copies, they are $8 each. Use the same procedure to request them. Once you receive the signed form back, your dissolution is final. You can find Hawaii laws online at: *www.capitol.hawaii.gov/*.

California Domestic Partnership

If you registered your domestic partnership with the state of California, the only way to dissolve the partnership is by following California procedures. If you have a California domestic partnership but do not live in California, you can terminate your partnership by mail if you meet certain requirements. If you live elsewhere and do not intend to return to California, you may decide there is no reason for you to file a termination in California. Note that it is unclear what effect a California dissolution order that includes property division will have on partners who live in another state.

If you registered your domestic partnership in California before the new and improved domestic partnerships law became effective in 2005, your partnership has been retroactively transformed into the newer version and the law applies to you.

There are two ways to terminate your California Domestic Partnership.

Secretary of State

The simplest way to terminate is through the California Secretary of State. You qualify only if you meet all of these criterion:

▼ You have both read the brochure available from the state. This form can be found at: *www.ss.ca.gov/dpregistrydp_faqs.htm#question8.*

▼ You both want to terminate the relationship.

▼ You have not been registered as California Domestic Partners for more than five years.

▼ No children were born to the two of you either before or during the domestic partnership.

▼ You did not adopt children during the domestic partnership.

▼ Neither of you is pregnant.

▼ Neither of you owns any land or buildings.

▼ Neither of you is renting land or buildings, except for your residence and if you rent for your residence, the lease does not include a purchase option and the lease will end within one year of the termination.

▼ Your community debt (incurred during your partnership), not including car loans, is less than $4,000.

▼ Your community property (property acquired during the partnership), not counting cars, is not worth more than $32,000.

▼ Not including cars, neither one of you has separate property worth more than $32,000.

▼ You have prepared and signed a property settlement agreement that describes how you will divide your assets and debts if you have community property and debts.

▼ Neither one of you wants support or money from the other beyond what you agreed to in your property settlement.

If you meet these requirements, you are eligible for this type of termination. To obtain your termination, file the form available at www.ss.ca.gov/dpregistry. You both must sign the form. The partnership will automatically be terminated six months after the date of filing. You each have the option of revoking the termination within this six month period, and your partnership will remain intact.

If you or your partner decides to revoke the termination, file a Notice of Revocation of Termination of Domestic Partnership with the California Secretary of State and send a copy to your partner by first class mail. Once you've revoked, you can't cancel the revocation. You will have to do a new termination if you wish to end the partnership.

You have no right to a hearing or appeal if you use this method of termination, but it is possible to have the termination set aside by a court in certain cases (such as if you didn't meet the eligibility requirements, were treated unfairly in the property settlement, or there are mistakes in the agreement).

Superior Court

If you aren't eligible for a simple termination through the Secretary of State's office, you must file a court proceeding with the California Superior Court. To begin, you must file a:

▼ Petition for Dissolution of Domestic Partnership (which gets you a dissolution, similar to a divorce).

▼ Petition for Judgment of Nullity of Domestic Partnership (which is similar to asking for annulment).

▼ Petition for Legal Separation of Domestic Partnership (which gives you a legal separation, so that you are still partners, but living apart).

The petition must be delivered to your partner by someone other than yourself. It takes about six months for a dissolution to make its way through the court process.

You can ask that the court send you to mediation to work out the issues before you, or you can decide to let the court make the decisions for you. You can also file the petition and file a copy of a settlement agreement you have reached on your own.

Custody

In California, you are both the legal parents of any children born to either of you or adopted by either of you during your partnership. When you dissolve your partnership, you need to make formal custody and child support arrangements.

The California Supreme Court has held that children born to a same sex couple (in this particular case, the case dealt with lesbians using insemination) are legal children of both partners, whether or not they have a domestic partnership agreement, and held that the parents have the duty to support the children. Based on this ruling, it is not necessary for a partner to adopt a child born to the other partner to obtain full legal parentage rights.

Property Division

California is a community property state and any assets or earnings acquired during the domestic partnership are considered community property and will be distributed in the dissolution. One interesting twist here though is that domestic partnerships are not covered by the spousal reassessment exemption that married couples have. A spousal reassessment exemption means that when you split up property, each spouse takes the asset and is not required to pay tax on it. Normally when you transfer an asset from one person to the other, tax has to be paid on the capital gains. Because domestic partnerships in California do not have this exemption, it is possible that the IRS could at some point subject these kinds of transfers to tax. To date this has not happened, but it is an important point to discuss with your attorney.

Legal Effect

If you relied on your domestic partnership to get benefits from a third party (such as health insurance through your partner's employer), you need to notify that party that the domestic partnership has been terminated within 60 days of the termination. A simple letter, sent registered mail, will be sufficient for this.

Getting Help

Forms are available online at *www.courtinfo.ca.gov*/forms To get a referral to an attorney in your county, see *www.dca.ca.gov/r_r/lawrefe1.htm*. To find a mediator, contact the Southern California Mediation Association at *www.scmediation.org* or the Northern California Mediation Center at *www.ncmc-mediate.org*, or look in your yellow pages under mediation to find one near you.

❖Kyle and Theo had a California domestic partnership and had been together for seven years. While they were together, Kyle adopted a baby girl from overseas. Theo did not officially adopt her. Their breakup was more of a growing apart than any big event. They didn't qualify for the Secretary of State dissolution and went to Superior Court. Because their daughter was adopted during the course of their partnership, Theo was also her legal parent and therefore custody and visitation had to be decided. They went to mediation and created a parenting plan that worked for both of them. The plan was incorporated by the court into the judgment of dissolution.

Chapter 6

Ending a Marriage That May Not Be Legal

If you were married in a city or county that allowed gay marriages for a brief period of time, you may be confused about whether or not your marriage is valid at this point. And if you're splitting up, you might decide you don't care. You do need to determine your legal status though. If your marriage is still valid, it means you can't marry or civil unionize with another future partner without a divorce. It also impacts your estate, tax status (depending on where you live), and responsibilities to each other.

This chapter sums up the current status of various localities at the time the book was written. However, this is an extremely fluid area of law right now with changes coming on a daily basis. You need to check to find out what your current status is before you make any decisions. To find out, contact Lambda Legal *www.lambdalegal.com* or your local pride or advocacy organization.

Additionally, there are several states where it is possible that gay marriage may become legal after this book is published. If you get married in a state not discussed in this book and decide you want a divorce but don't know how to go about it, start with the state court system Website. Often, do-it-yourself forms for divorce are available there. If you are allowed to "marry," you can use your state's regular divorce forms. If the state legalizes something else, such as a domestic partnership or a civil union, there may be different forms, so check with Lambda Legal, your state advocacy organization, or just go in and ask the court clerk for help. If you are married in a location not discussed in this chapter (things are changing quickly, so it is possible that some localities may offer licenses and later have them questioned or voided), but are uncertain as to the legality of the marriage, check with the local court system or Lambda Legal for information about the status of your marriage.

San Francisco, California

At the time this book was written, San Francisco marriages were still being appealed. If you were married here and break up, you first need to find out the current status of the case (see the previous suggestions or check the *San Francisco Chronicle* online at *www.sfgate.com/ chronicle/* for breaking news). Things have been changing quickly, so you may be married one day and not the next. The best plan may be to ride things out and see how the courts resolve this. Don't go through the time, effort, and expense of ending a marriage that may ultimately be held invalid. Once things are final though, if the marriages are upheld, you will need to get a divorce. You can get information and forms about California divorce online at *www.courtinfo.ca.gov/selfhelp/family/ divorce/*.

❖Kal and Tom were married in San Francisco, where they lived. Unfortunately, Tom fell in love with someone else and wants a divorce. Kal took the news hard, but is determined to get on with his life and is sure there is someone else out there for him that will make him happy. Tom is now living with his new partner and would like to get married, or at least register a domestic partnership. Tom went to see an attorney, who advised him that he should just try to wait and see what happens with the legality of his marriage. The attorney pointed out that if the marriages are held invalid, Tom will have spent a lot of money on a divorce that wasn't necessary. Tom really wanted to move forward with his new partner, but they talked it over and agreed that it just made more sense to wait and see what happened. In the meantime, Tom has revoked all of his existing legal documents that involve Kal and has executed new ones with his new partner.

Multnomah County, Oregon

Multnomah marriages have been held invalid by the state, so if you were married in Oregon, your marriage is no longer valid. You don't need to do anything to end your partnership, unless you executed documents as partners, or have joint assets and debts (see Chapter 9 for information about how to deal with this).

New York State

If you were married in one of the several cities or towns in New York State that did same sex marriages, your status is currently up in the air at the time this book was written.

Note that under New York law, you do not need a valid marriage license to be considered legally married. If you were married in a marriage ceremony by an authorized official, your marriage is legal. So even if you were not issued a marriage license (as those married in New Paltz were not), your marriage is legal as long as the New York state courts hold that same sex marriage is legal in the state, if the legislature passes a gay marriage law, or until New York courts decide these marriages are not legal. It's important to note that even though these marriages are technically legal, they are probably not recognized as such by many, including court clerks and other government employees.

Additionally, there is some confusion over New York officially recognizing same sex unions. The state attorney general issued an opinion that New York should recognize same sex unions from other states in the same way it recognizes New York marriages. Based on this opinion, and the legal background behind it, it is possible that same sex married couples may be able to get a divorce in New York, using New York divorce procedures. The answer won't be certain until there is a test case.

If you wish to seek a New York divorce, forms and information are available online at *www.courts.state.ny.us/ courthelp*. For legal assistance in the state of New York, contact the lawyer referal program at *www.nysba.org/ Template.cfm?Section=Lawyer_Referral* or (800) 342-3661.

Sandoval County, New Mexico

If you obtained a marriage license in Sandoval County and were married, your marriage is not legal at this time. The state declared licenses issued here invalid. If you executed documents giving each other legal authority, see Chapter 9.

Chapter 7

Ending a Partnership Under Contract

If you are one of many couples that are not legally joined but who have created their own partnership agreements, you may be unsure of what to do now that your relationship has ended and uncertain as to what impact your partnership agreement has now.

Types of Agreements

There are a wide variety of domestic partnership agreements and contracts, so there is no one answer for how your contract or agreement will affect your breakup.

Some couples have loosely-written guidelines for their lives together, which may not even be signed. This is essentially an oral agreement. The best way to handle an oral agreement is to talk to each other calmly and try to work out a plan for the division of assets and debts.

Other couples have signed contracts that lay out their rights and responsibilities in a clear-cut manner. Some other partners have an agreement that is somewhere in between the two previously discussed. It might be in writing and signed, but it is rather rough and with few details.

No matter what kind of agreement you have, it is possible to end your relationship in a reasonable and fair way. You should sit down and look at your agreement together and see if there is a way to honor it. If you both agree to make some changes to it, that's okay, too, as long as you both agree. It may be best to put these changes into writing, so that it is clear what you agreed to and also so it is clear that you have modified the terms of the original agreement.

What to Do if Only One Person Wants Out

If you are not in agreement about ending your partnership, this can't stop one person from picking up and leaving. There is nothing you do to stop a breakup. If one of you doesn't follow the terms of your contract, you can try to convince him or her otherwise, ask a friend to intervene, convince the other partner to go to mediation, or as a last alternative, go to court.

Contract Terms and Enforceability

Just because you have something in writing does not mean that it will be upheld by a court. Unless your contract has a severability clause in it, if one contract provision is found to be invalid, the entire contract is thrown out and can't be considered. This is a common problem if you wrote up the agreement yourselves. If you had an attorney draw up a domestic partnership agreement, it's most likely going to be enforceable.

For a contract to be legally enforceable there has to be what is called "consideration." You each must receive some benefit from the contract. If you agreed to pay your partner $500 a month and in exchange you shared the apartment that is in her name, you have received a benefit from your agreement. If however you agreed to pay your partner $500 a month, but got nothing in return, there would be no consideration.

For a contract to be valid there has to be offer and acceptance, meaning both of you have to agree to the terms of the contract. If one of you wrote up a contract and gave it to the other, but the other partner didn't actually agree to the contract, it isn't valid.

If a contract is signed under duress (force) then it is not valid. Also, if one party in the contract did not have all the information at the time of signing, it will not be valid. So, for example, if a couple signed a co-habitation agreement and in it was a provision that partner A would receive no more than $5,000 from partner B if they break up, and partner A thought partner B had little or no income or property, when in fact he owned a huge company and earned hundreds of thousands of dollars, this would be an instance in which partner A did not have all the facts.

Contract terms that have to do with financial things such as money and property, as well as debts, are enforceable. Agreements about custody or visitation would not be immediately enforceable because you need a judge's approval and a court order. For a discussion of spousal support enforceability, see Chapter 12. Sometimes partners include things in their agreements that aren't enforceable by courts. These are mainly lifestyle issues such as who will take out the trash or that one partner will stay home and care for the children. Courts are only going to enforce clear-cut provisions that deal with property, assets, or debts.

The best way to avoid questions of enforceability is to avoid going to court at all costs. Try to work something out on your own. Some agreement is better than none and if you go to court you may find that your entire agreement is invalid.

How to End Your Partnership Agreement

If you and your partner agree about the terms in your contract, or if you agree to divide your property and debts in some other way, there is no problem. If you both agree, you can do anything you want. To end your partnership, when you agree for the most part, you don't need to do anything formal in a legal sense. Divide your property and debts (see chapter 9 for more information). If you have children, consult chapters 10 and 11. Take care of your business and go your separate ways.

If you disagree about what your agreement says, you may need help working through your breakup. Read about your type of agreement and suggested remedies:

Oral or Informal Agreement

If you have an oral or informal agreement, it is important that you try to work out a settlement together. Nobody wants to go to court, and if you have an oral or informal agreement, it is very difficult to prove what you agreed to, or if there even was an agreement at all. Each person may have a different take on what was really agreed to (and this may not be deception—you might truly have each understood things in a different way).

If you disagree about what you previously agreed to, or how it should be interpreted, consider sitting down together and each presenting a written breakdown of how you believe the issues between you should be handled. You may find that you agree on quite a few things. Then try to seek a compromise on each of the issues you disagree over. If you are still unable to come to terms, consider asking a mutual friend to sit with both of you and try to sort it out. If this fails, consider seeing a mediator (see Chapter 13). If mediation does not work, you are left with small claims court as your only option. You will need to prove to the judge that you and your partner had an agreement, that the terms were clear and understood, that you both consented to them, and that your partner has failed to follow the terms of the agreement.

Written Agreement That Is Vague

If you do have a written and signed agreement, but the terms of it are not clear, you and your partner will need to discuss how you will interpret those sections. When you wrote it you probably had some sense of what you intended. It's time now to sit down and discuss that and try to come to an understanding. If you can't agree, try having a friend help or use mediation. Court should be your last resort. Even though you have something in writing, it is vague and will be open to interpretation. The judge will rely on oral testimony from each of you to determine what you thought these sections meant when you signed the agreement. In the end, it is little better than an oral agreement because the interpretation depends on your testimony.

Clear Written Agreement

If you have a clear written contract signed by both of you, and you're squabbling over it, your best bet is to either recognize that you've got to live by the terms of the contract, or reach a mutually agreeable compromise. If your contract is clear and concise, a judge is simply going to apply its terms. It is a waste of your time to try to argue otherwise, unless you and your partner entered in a later written or oral agreement that somehow changed or affected the terms of your partnership agreement.

Follow these steps during a breakup when you have a contract:

▼ Read your contract and see what it says about ending your relationship.

▼ Decide if you feel the contract is enforceable.

▼ Decide if you want to abide by the terms of the agreement or if you feel it isn't fair or is unclear or unenforceable.

▼ Talk with your partner about the contract and try to create a plan you both agree on. If you can't agree, ask a friend to help you.

▼ If a friend can't help or doesn't want to get involved, see a mediator.

▼ If mediation fails, try again to reach an agreement on your own.

▼ Consider how important the items you are disputing are to you.

▼ If you can't let it go, file a small claims case or see an attorney.

❖Ann and Vanessa wrote a partnership agreement together when they committed to each other. In it they outlined how they would share expenses and income and set up some rules for the ways they would organize certain things—such as Vanessa was responsible for writing the checks for all the bills and Ann was in charge of the grocery

continued on next page

shopping. They also agreed that should they break up, they would evenly divide all joint property and each would keep the property she came into the relationship with. They agreed that they would equally be responsible for household debts. Despite some couples counseling, they ended their relationship.

It seemed as though they were going to be able to manage the financial aspect of their breakup without any problems, until Ann's mother convinced her that there was no reason why she should pay half of the credit card bill for the kayak Vanessa was keeping. Ann also cleaned out their joint bank account. Vanessa was stunned. Although she no longer wanted to be with Ann, she couldn't believe Ann would treat her this way. She asked Ann repeatedly to follow the terms of their agreement. Ann refused to talk to a mutual friend or go to mediation. Vanessa was going back to school and really needed the money she believed Ann owed her; so she filed a case in small claims court. She found some of the paperwork confusing and felt sick the night she had to go in and testify.

Testifying turned out not to be so hard. Ann showed up and tried to twist things, but Vanessa had their agreement, as well as official records from the bank and credit card company that the court clerk helped her obtain. The judge told them that their contract was not enforceable because there were too many provisions in it that could not be upheld by a court. However, he ruled that there was a clear oral agreement between the two of them about how their debts and property would be divided. He ordered Ann
continued on next page

to pay Vanessa the amount she was asking for. Vanessa was really relieved.

Two months later, she wasn't feeling so relieved. Ann still hadn't paid. Vanessa called the court and asked what she could do. She was going to have to file more papers and go back to court and ask the judge to hold Ann in contempt of court for not paying the money and ask that her wages be garnished or her bank account attached. Vanessa decided she just couldn't go through all that again and so she decided to just let it go. She's not sure she made the right decision, but thinks that for now, it's what works for her.

How to Use Small Claims Court

If you and your partner cannot work out an agreement on your own or with the help of a mediator or friend, you are left with small claims court as your only avenue. You should avoid this whenever possible, but in some cases, there is simply no other choice. If your partner is refusing to divide a substantial amount of money or pay his or her share of a debt, small claims court is an option you have no choice but to pursue.

Small claims courts can be found in every town and municipality. Look in the government pages of your phone book or call your town hall to find out where the court is located. Go in to see the court clerk and ask for the forms you need to file a small claims case. Each town has its own forms and most towns will provide you with an instruction booklet as well, outlining your rights and the procedures. Or you can access forms and instructions online through your state judiciary Website (do a search for the name of your state and the words *judiciary* or *courts*). Ask what the jurisdictional limit is. This is the highest amount of money the court is allowed to deal with. So if your small claims court has a limit of $5,000 but you want to sue your ex for $10,000, you must either decide to go to the next highest level of court in your area (state or county) or sue only for the maximum amount you can get in small claims court.

Small claims cases are handled relatively quickly and may be in front of a judge or jury. You don't need an attorney and the court is very flexible with unrepresented (pro se) parties. You'll file your papers and will most likely have a preliminary appearance where the judge will ask you if you can reach a settlement. If you can't, a date will be set for the trial. You can call witnesses, including anyone who has first hand knowledge of your agreement. You can present evidence, such as a written contract (you'll need the original), bank account statements, and credit card bills. You have the opportunity to testify and tell your side of the story and the chance to cross-examine your partner about what he or she has to say. Usually only an hour or so will be allotted for your trial.

Once the judge makes a decision, an order or judgment will be issued, explaining what he or she has decided. This is the final decision and you have to follow it. You always have the right to appeal, however it is important to understand that an appeal only looks at whether the judge applied the law correctly, not what the facts of the case were. If you want to appeal, ask the court clerk what papers you need to file.

Chapter 8

Ending a Nonformalized Relationship

There are many couples who live in states where there is no legal way to formalize their union and who see no need to write up a contract. If you're in this group, you might feel as if there is no help available to you or laws that govern your situation. You do have rights though, and it is important to understand what they are.

Issues With Children

It's important to remember that if you have children and you are both legal parents, your state's family court will make custody and visitation arrangements for you, or approve a settlement you come up with. However, you still need to go to court and get an order even if you are in agreement. Child support is also handled in family court. Family court is available to any parents, no matter what sex they are or whether they are married to each other or not. You'll have to go to family court to get your custody and visitation arrangements made official. See Chapter 11 for more information about this.

Your Rights

When your relationship ends, you're thinking about how you're going to recover, but you're also stuck dealing with the mechanics of who is going to take the peace lily and who is going to pay the cable bill. When you have no agreement with each other at all about how these things are going to happen, you might feel confused as to how you should handle things.

You should each take the things that belonged to you before you moved in together and things you purchased separately for yourselves. Then you've got to find a way to divide up those things that are joint property. You also probably have some debts and while they are probably in separate names, you may know that you're each responsible for them in part. You'll need to work out a plan for how you can divide responsibility for these debts. See Chapter 9 for information and assistance in dividing up property and debts.

If you can't work   anything out, try mediation and settlement talks. If you can't work out something that way, you'll find yourselves in court (see page 106-107 for a description of small claims court procedures), or you'll find yourselves walking away with no resolution at all. If you think you can live with things as they've been left, you may have no reason to go court. But if there are some things that absolutely have to be resolved, court is your only option if mediation and self-negotiation fails.

But what are you rights? How will a court decide what to do for you? Any property or debt either one of you came into the relationship with, you'll leave with. Items that you bought together or are in both of your names will be totaled and each of you will be entitled to part of the total value. This can be accomplished either by one person paying the other one, or by dividing up the property so that you each walk away with things of equal value. Who gets how much will be determined by how much you each contributed to the cost of the item and what your promises were to each other about it.

If you have debts that have both your names on it, such as a lease, utility bill, credit card bill, and so on, you'll each be responsible for half the amount due, unless you can show that you had some agreement otherwise. If you have debts that are in one person's name, but were intended to be joint (such as if you went grocery shopping and put the bill on your credit card, or you took a trip to Florida and put the airfare on your partner's card), you'll have to prove to the court that one person took out the debt as a way to give a loan to the other. For example, you paid for the groceries with the understanding that your partner was supposed to pay you for his or her half later. These kinds of determinations can be very difficult for a court to make and very difficult for you as a litigant to prove. There's no question that part of the hurdle you'll be facing is the fact that some small claims court judges are just not used to hearing cases dealing with the division of assets and debts from gay or lesbian partners. Additionally, these judges are not skilled at handling these kinds of cases because heterosexuals with these issues go to family or divorce court.

What if Only One Person Wants Out?

If only one of you wants the relationship to end, the person leaving can access all joint bank accounts and remove funds (although a court might decide that he or she took more than his/her share and has to pay some of it back). He or she would also be able to remove any separate property.

If he or she wanted to remove joint property and the other partner was against it, your best bet is to try and work out some kind of compromise. Calling the police will not help because you both have an equal right to the items and traditionally the police have not been very helpful in this kind of dispute. A court could decide that the property should not have been taken, but even if the court rules this way, getting your ex to give it back is another matter entirely.

❖Dan and Tim lived together for two years. They had no written agreement and had not registered a partnership or formalized their relationship. When they moved in together, they both felt it was something they would take day-by-day.

After two years it became clear that they just weren't right for each other. Their interests and goals were just too different and they found themselves fighting all the time. They split the grocery costs each month. Each bought his own clothes and personal belongings. They had a joint bank account they used for household expenses. Each contributed part of his salary to that account each month. While they were together they purchased stereo equipment, a new refrigerator, and lots of Christmas decorations.

When Tim decided to move out, there was $2,000 in the joint bank account after that month's bills. They both had ideas about how they felt things should be divided up. It made sense to both of them that Dan keep the refrigerator because he would be remaining in the apartment. After some discussion they agreed Tim would take the sound system. They both felt very emotional about the Christmas

continued on next page

decorations and decided the best way to handle it was just to get it all out and take turns selecting things. Once they got to talking about the money, things were a little more difficult. Tim felt that because Dan was keeping the refrigerator, that he ought to take the money in the account. Tim disagreed because they each contributed equally to that account. Dan ended up leaving without getting the money issue resolved. A few days later he called and suggested that he take three fourths of the money and Tim take the remaining fourth. Tim wasn't too pleased about this. He suggested that if Dan gave him the upholstered bench that fit so perfectly underneath the window in the hall, which was Dan's before they moved in together, that he would do it. They agreed and were able to split fairly amicably.

Chapter 9

Dividing Your Property and Debts

Dividing up property is the one thing that is common to the end of all relationships. No matter whether you were married, civil unioned, in a domestic partnership, or any other kind of relationship, you and your partner shared a home or residence, property, and debts. When you break up, dividing all of it up can be a difficult task.

How you divide your property and debts will in part be controlled by what kind of partnership you had. If you had a marriage or civil union, you can divide them in any way you agree on as long as it is approved by the court, but if you ask a judge to do it, he or she will make decisions based on that state's laws. If you have a contract or co-habitation agreement, you will need to either follow the terms of that contract, or agree on an alternate method of dividing property and debt. The bottom line is you can do just about anything you want if you both agree.

If you can't agree, and your state has no divorce or dissolution procedure available to you, your only other option is to use mediation, or go to small claims court. (See Chapter 7 for tips on using small claims court.)

Coping With Property and Debt Division

Property and debt division is a difficult thing to deal with. For most people it's about more than deciding who gets the double boiler and who gets the wok. We assign emotional values to our property. There are memories and feelings attached to items. The division of property also, for many people, becomes symbolic of their relationship or their feelings for each other. Getting more stuff sometimes seems to equal winning or being proven right. Holding on to certain items can be a way of holding on to the relationship, or a way of avoiding facing the next step in your life.

The key to dividing up property smoothly is to remember it's just stuff. And you can always buy more stuff. You've got to look at your property division rationally. Is it the end of the world if you take 10 DVDs instead of 15? You have to remember that neither one of you is going to walk away from this whole. You can't take the stuff from one household and split it in half and have enough to comfortably furnish and equip two households. It is simply not possible. So you're both going to end up buying things once this is over.

When you're breaking up it's easy to let discussions about property division and money get out of hand. There are complicated issues of fairness, equality, and need mixed up with the emotional issues mentioned earlier. Keeping your head screwed on straight is going to be difficult, but it's the only way you're going to get through this. You've got to approach it in a rational way. Essentially what you're doing is a business deal—a financial transaction. If you try to treat it as though it is a business agreement, you'll be able to stay cool and not get so emotional (at least not in the moment—go ahead and cry and scream before or afterwards).

❖Laura and Whitney were splitting up and were having terrible fights about their property division. Whitney changed her mind every day about what she wanted. Laura would think she knew what she wanted but then she would talk to Whitney and go into a complete tailspin and not know what to do. Neither of them was willing to move out until they figured out who got what because neither trusted the other. Each night they would come home and start on each other. It was completely unbearable. Finally Laura had lunch with an old friend, Tammy, who had recently ended her heterosexual marriage. Laura confided in Tammy about what was going on and Tammy explained how she and her ex had managed to work out a settlement on their own without any help. Tammy told her to get organized and make a list of everything they needed to decide and then e-mail Whitney and set up an "appointment" for the coming weekend to sit down and work things out. She suggested that Laura include a list of rules they could follow at their meeting that might help them stay on track. Laura tried it and Whitney agreed to the meeting. It wasn't easy and it took several sessions, but they were finally able to work something out that they were both satisfied with.

Separate Property

Separate property is anything you owned before you lived together including any gifts, inheritances, or personal injury settlement awards you received during the relationship. If you're not married/civil unioned (or you are dissolving your marriage in a state other than one that recognized marriages or civil unions) items you purchased separately during the relationship are also separate property.

If one of you owns a piece of separate property, but the non owner spouse did something to improve the value of the property (such as doing home repairs or doing body work on a car), then he or she jointly owns the increase in value on that property.

Separate Debts

Debts that you had when you entered into the relationship remain separate. Debts incurred during the relationship that have both names on them are a joint responsibility. Debts incurred during the relationship in one name are considered joint if you're married or civil unioned. In other states, if the debt was incurred to benefit both of you (for example a credit card bill to buy a plasma screen television you both used and considered joint), then a court may direct the unlisted partner to pay a portion of it.

How to Divide Property

The best way to divide property is to first focus on need. There is no sense in you taking the lawn mower if you're moving into a condo. If your partner is a graphic designer, she probably has more use for the computer than you do if you're a landscaper. Once you've divided up the things that one person needs but the other one probably doesn't, you can look at ways to divide up the rest. The following are some tips for household property division:

▼ Keep sets together. China, collections, matching furniture, and so on all have more value when they remain intact.

▼ Don't take things out of spite. You may have always hated the Queen Anne coffee table, but suddenly when you're breaking up, getting it will signify a win for you. Take only things you want and will really use.

▼ Don't be afraid to sell some things and split the cash. If neither of you is going to use the dining room set, get rid of it and get cash that you can both use.

▼ Keep children's items with the children. If your kids will be spending more time at one house than the other, it makes sense that most of their stuff would go to that house.

▼ Focus on use, not value. It's best to divide items up according to who will use it. You can total it all up and look at the bottom line value of what you each got and make adjustments with cash or investments to compensate if necessary.

▼ Remember you are going to have a new life. Your life will change after the divorce, so you may find your needs are vastly different now than they were. Take the things that support your new lifestyle.

You and your spouse should plan a time to have a property division meeting. Before you sit down and talk about this, make some lists. List the things you must have—these are not negotiable. Then list the things you think you really don't want at all. Next list the things you think you want, but may be willing to negotiate over. Then when you and your partner sit down, create a new list and write down each item and who is getting it. You can also estimate each item's value so that you will be able to come up with a total value for each of you. There will be things you don't agree on immediately. Set these things aside or write them on your list with a question mark after them. Try to work out some trades, such as, "you can take the vacuum if I get the weed whacker." You can also make trade offs with debt or cash, such as, "I want the treadmill and if you let me have it, I'll pay this month's electric bill." Be creative and try to think outside the box. Your partner might agree to let you take the lawn furniture if you agree to give him the Burberry coat that you own but you both wore on occasion.

Once you've divided things up as best you can, total up approximate values and see how the bottom line is looking. Then do your division of cash, investments, and debts with this in mind. If one of you is coming out ahead in property division, it might make sense for the other to take less cash or more debt.

Being Realistic

It's also important to be realistic about property division. Do you really want to itemize every mug, pair of socks, and deck of cards? Probably not. Focus on the big stuff when you're making lists and let the small stuff happen naturally (one of you moves out and packs some of it up and goes).

It can be easy to get caught up in trying to make things come out completely even. If you are both happy with the way you've divided things, don't get hung up on bottom line value. Remember that the actual value of household items is hard to pinpoint because it might be worth a lot to you but may not be something you could actually sell for very much.

How to Divide Debt

Dividing up your debts is even less fun than dividing property because no one wants to be responsible for a debt if they can help it. You may want to divide up your debts when you divide your assets—debts that are related to assets could go to the person getting that asset. So if you take the car, you take the car loan. Other debts such as credit card debts can be divided in half, or you could prorate them based on your separate incomes.

When considering debt, be sure to at least consider the following:

▼ Mortgages.

▼ Leases and unpaid rent.

▼ Home equity loans.

▼ Personal/unsecured loans.

▼ Student loans.

▼ Lines of credit (overdraft).

▼ Loans against life insurance.

▼ Loans from friends and family.

▼ Loans against retirement or pension accounts.

▼ Credit cards.

▼ Unpaid utilities.

▼ Unpaid health care costs.

▼ Installment payments.

Negotiating

Remember that dividing up property and debt is about negotiation. You may want to play some cards close to the vest. For example, don't tell your partner you really don't want the Kitchen Aid mixer or the big screen TV, and use them as bargaining chips to get the sleigh bed.

Remember that negotiations can take time and you might need to have a couple of meetings to really sort everything out.

If you're having a hard time getting through this together, consider asking a friend to help you work it out. If that doesn't work, mediation is a good choice.

How to Divide Certain Things

Real Estate

When thinking about real estate, you need to be aware of the legal constraints. If you are renters and both of your names are on the lease and only one of you will remain there, you need to get a new lease issued in one name. If you don't, you both continue to be legally responsible for the rent. So if partner A stays and partner B leaves, but partner A skips out on the rent, the landlord can come after partner B for the money.

If only one person's name is on the lease and the non-named party will be staying, he or she will have to sublet or else the landlord will need to issue a new lease in his or her name.

If you live in a home or apartment that you jointly own, you can do a quit claim deed transferring ownership to one partner. The mortgage however is another matter (see later in this chapter for information). If only one name is on the title and the nonowner will keep the property, you need to make a sale of the property and consult an attorney.

❖Emilio and Taz had lived together in Emilio's house for five years. Taz was a skilled carpenter and during that time he installed new kitchen cabinets,
continued on next page

opened up the dining room so it connected to the kitchen and built a deck. When they broke up, they both knew that Emilio would keep the house because it was his originally, even though they both felt that in some ways it had come to belong to both of them. Taz pointed out that he had done a lot of work on the house which had increased its value significantly and felt that when they divided their property that he ought to be compensated. Emilio knew that this was fair but he wasn't sure how to decide what the work was worth. His brother's girlfriend was an attorney and she pointed out that he should get the house appraised and compare it to what it was worth when he bought it the year before Taz moved in. He did that and he and Taz agreed to apply half of the increase in value as having come from the renovations (and the other half from appreciation over time). To compensate for this, they transferred a mutual fund account from joint names to Taz's name. The account was worth $12,000, but because it was in joint names, only half the value was considered a gift from Emilio to Taz and there was no gift tax.

Vehicles

To transfer vehicle ownership, check your state DMV Website for information about on how to transfer a title. You may have to make a "sale" in order to transfer from one partner to the other in a state where there is no gay marriage.

Bank Accounts and Investments

If you have joint accounts, either of you can remove funds at any time. You'll want to get these joint accounts closed, to prevent potential problems with one of you emptying them without agreement. If you have joint investments, you may want to roll them over into individual accounts or simply pay one partner cash in exchange for changing the account to an individual account. Note that this is something you'll need to be sure to discuss with your tax preparer because you may have capital gains taxes to deal with for investments. Also see the discussion later in this chapter about gift tax.

Retirement Accounts

If you live in a state that recognizes your marriage or union, you can transfer ownership of retirement accounts as part of your divorce. In other states you can't transfer these accounts, but you can give one partner cash (or other property) as compensation for his or her interest in an account the other partner holds (but again, be sure to understand gift tax law).

Pets

For many people, pets are more than just a kind of property. It can be hard to work out which partner a beloved pet will live with, but it's important to remember that you can always work out a time-sharing agreement or visitation plan so that the pet has time with both of you. You will want to consider what the pet's needs are (for example a golden retriever needs a lot of exercise) and what each of your schedules and lifestyles will be like once you're living apart. It's also possible to work out an arrangement that allows you to share the pet's expenses, such as veterinary care, licensing, dog walking, grooming, and medications.

Businesses

If you jointly own a business together, you can either arrange a buyout by one partner or work out some kind of arrangement that allows you to continue together as owners. You must consider your own individual situation to know what will work for you.

If you are going to arrange a buyout, you may need to get the business valued so that you each understand what it is really worth. A buyout can happen all at once or payments can be made over a period of time. Be sure to consult an attorney to help you make the buyout legal.

If one of you owns a business and the other has done things to add to the value of that business during the course of your relationship, he or she may be entitled to something to compensate him or her for this. If you live in a state where marriages are legal, there will be established case law that determines how the business and the contributions are measured.

Credit Card Debts

If you have joint credit card debts, you need to either pay them off or transfer the balances off to individual accounts. If you have any credit cards in your name for which your spouse is an authorized user, remove his or her name from the account.

If there are individual credit card accounts that have balances on them for things you agree are joint, you can't transfer the balance to the other partner's account. One spouse can pay the other one for his or her share of that debt.

If you don't agree about debts on individual cards, first try having a friend help you try to reach a solution.

Next try mediation. If you can't get anywhere, you have a choice of either walking away from it or going to court. If you are in a state where your marriage is recognized, individual credit cards are considered marital debt, and so you must divide these as part of your property and debt settlement. If your state does not recognize your marriage, then you would need to prove that the debt was intended to be joint and that you both received a benefit from it.

Mortgages

If you have a joint mortgage or home equity loan, there is no way to remove one spouse's name from the mortgage (even if a court determines only one of you is going to be responsible for the debt) because the court has no jurisdiction over the bank. There is also no way to transfer part of the balance of the mortgage. The only way to change a mortgage is to refinance it. So if one of you will be keeping the home and will take on the mortgage, you must refinance it into that partner's name alone. You can work out a trade with other assets and debts to compensate the partner who is taking on the mortgage. Again, be aware of gift tax implications.

It is possible to continue owning real estate and having a mortgage together after you break up and some couples continue to successfully own rental properties together, but in most situations this does not work well.

Special Kinds of Property

There are some other assets you should think about that may not seem so obvious. If one of you got a degree or a professional license during the course of your relationship and the other partner worked, supported you, or made sacrifices in order for you to do that, a divorce court would consider the value of that license or degree to be marital property.

Gym memberships, frequent flyer miles, credit card points, and other nontangible assets might be in joint names, or have one person's name on it and really belong to both of you. A divorce court would consider these things to be marital assets. Just because a divorce court would divide these things up does not mean you have to, but these are types of property you should be aware of when you are negotiating.

Budgeting

Once you have an idea of how you and your partner want to divide things, you need to think about what your budget is going to be like after you complete your divorce. If you live in a state where you have a formal divorce process available to you, you will need to present the court with a budget as part of your financial disclosure process. A budget can help you understand exactly what you've agreed to take on and help you think about how your income compares to your expenses. The budget can help you get a grip on what your financial life is going to look like post-divorce and help you realize now if you've taken on more debt than you can manage or if you need to find a higher paying job.

Gift Tax Concerns

If you and your partner are not married in the eyes of your state, you need to be careful when you transfer property to each other—whether it is separately owned or joint. You each own half the value of joint property and so if you transfer an investment account from joint names to your name alone, it could be considered that your partner has given you a gift on his or her behalf. However, you can give gifts of up to $11,000 per year per person without triggering gift tax. You can also pay educational or medical expenses for anyone without it being considered a gift, as long as you pay the money directly to the school or health care provider.

Chapter 10

Children and Divorce

If there are children in your relationship, your divorce is painful and difficult for them as well, no matter who their legal parents are. It is important to remember that children grow emotionally attached to parents—legal parents are important, but what matters to a child is the relationship he or she has with adults in his or her life. Even if the child is not a legal child of one of you, he or she has bonded to that person and created a parent-child attachment. There are ways to work out arrangements so that both of you continue to have a relationship with your children, even if there seems to be no legal support.

Legal and Emotional Parents

Custody laws only deal with legal parents. If you and your partner are not both legal parents, there is no court that is going to award visitation to the no legal parent. You are in essence a stepparent and stepparents have no legal right to seek custody or visitation. In a stepparent situation, it is completely up to the two of you to take steps to allow the child to maintain that important parent-child connection.

A legal parent must either have physically given birth to the child, been married to (or civil unioned to) the child's mother when the child was born, or legally adopted the child. In California, if one partner gives birth to the child, the other partner is the legal parent even if there is no formal domestic partnership. A legal parent is the only one who has any standing in a court of law to request custody or visitation.

An emotional parent is a person who has filled a parental role in the child's life and has a bond with him or her. If you and your partner lived together in the same house and parented together, you are both emotional parents. It is important to point out that children can have more than two emotional parents. If your ex-husband is the child's father and he still has a relationship with your child, then you, your partner, and your ex-husband are all emotional parents. And if your ex-husband remarries, his new wife may become an emotional parent as well. Having a lot of emotional parents is not harmful—it just provides your child with a larger support system.

If you and your partner have not been together long, then it is possible that whoever is not the legal parent may not have developed a very strong bond with the child—and that's okay, too. But recognize that any time a person is important in your life, that person carries some importance in your child's life and therefore the separation cannot be painless. It's important for you and your partner to take a look at what kind of relationship exists with the child and think about the best way to continue that relationship.

Helping Your Child

The most important thing is to be honest with your child. Don't downplay what is happening or lie to him. Saying that your partner is going away for a while when in fact he or she is moving out permanently will just confuse your child. Sit down with your child together, if possible, and tell him or her that the two of you have decided not to live together anymore. You do not need to provide details about why you've decided this, but you can offer general explanations such as "we don't love each other anymore," or "we aren't happy together." Read some books about children and divorce to help you understand how your child may react, or the questions he or she may ask.

It is absolutely essential that you explain to your child that you both love her and always will. Explain that while adults can sometimes stop loving each other, parents never stop loving their kids. If one of you is not a legal parent, be sure to point out to the child that the two of them will continue to see each other and do things together. Your child needs to know that one parental figure is not just going to disappear. Offer your child a concrete schedule for how you will share time. Take the time to answer questions your child has and expect your child to come up with questions over a long period of time about this.

There are some relationships in which the nonlegal parent does not want to have an ongoing relationship with the child, particularly if the marriage was brief and if the child was the product of an earlier heterosexual marriage. In this case, the first thing to do is to try and convince the nonlegal parent to keep in touch with the child somehow. If you can't manage that, then explain honestly to your child that you simply don't know when she'll see your partner again, but be certain to point out that none of this is a reflection on her, and is instead a part of the turmoil between adults.

Expect your child to go through a range of emotions over the divorce—anger, blame, insecurity, fear, regression, sadness, and depression. It takes a long time to adjust to such a big change in family life, and if your child is changing residences, it can take even longer.

Follow these do's and don'ts to help your child get through this difficult time.

DO:

▼ Make it clear that you will both be a part of his or her life.

▼ Repeat how much you both love him or her and will always be there for her.

▼ Help him or her understand the logistics— who will be where, when.

▼ Present things as a done deal. Make it clear there will be no reconciliation.

▼ Encourage his or her relationship with the other parent.

▼ Be patient with your child and give him or her some time to process everything that is going on.

▼ Answer his or her questions in an honest, age appropriate way.

▼ Let your child know the divorce is not his or her fault and he had nothing to do with it.

▼ Make yourself available to talk about the divorce as your child processes through it.

▼ Do things together as a family at times if it is comfortable. Some parents include their ex at birthday parties or holidays.

DON'T:

▼ Use your child as your therapist. He or she doesn't need to hear all the details of your emotional life.

▼ Use your child as a messenger. Asking your child to carry messages, either oral or written, places him or her directly in the center of whatever conflict is going on. As the adults, it is your responsibility to communicate with each other and not use your child as a buffer.

▼ Say negative things about your ex in front of your child. Allow him or her to maintain positive feelings about the other person.

▼ Use your child as a spy. Whatever goes on at your ex's house is none of your business, unless it puts your child in danger.

▼ Pretend that the other parent no longer exists. Even if there is no legal tie there, there is still an emotional bond.

Getting Help for Your Child

You've got a lot on your plate trying to deal with your own reactions to the divorce. Helping your child through it can be a challenge. If you think that you want to get some outside help for your child, there are lots of avenues. If your child is in school, consider talking to the school social worker. He or she can meet with your child and provide some support. Some schools have group meetings for kids whose parents are divorcing. Letting the social worker know can also be important if your child's teacher is not sensitive to your family's situation.

There are many excellent therapists who can give your child a safe place to talk and offer coping strategies. To find a therapist, ask your pediatrician for a referral, or contact your health insurance company for a list of names that participate in your plan. Make sure any therapist you use is licensed by your state and experienced in helping children deal with divorce. If possible, try to stick to a therapist who specializes in children and one who has worked with children of gay families.

Banana Splits is a national school-based program that offers support and peer assistance for kids experiencing divorce. Ask your school social worker or contact the program's national office at: Banana Splits, 53 Columbus Avenue #2, New York, NY 10023. Or call them at (212) 262-4562.

Legal Parents

If you are the legal parent, it is not advisable for you to put any agreement about your arrangements with the nonlegal parent in writing. Even though you are willing to make room in your child's life for a relationship with the other parent, you do not want to provide any evidence that could later be used in court to suggest you are giving up parental rights in any way to your former partner.

If you are not the legal parent, a written schedule gives you a firmer agreement, even if you are not looking to try and obtain custody someday.

Using a Court to Decide Custody

If you and your partner are both legal parents, you can file a petition in your local family court, (and you must go to court, even if it is just to present your settlement to the court) asking the judge to decide custody and visitation. You don't need an attorney to do this. Family court is usually designed to be user-friendly and the court personnel can help you complete the necessary forms. You can go straight to family court if you and your partner disagree, or if you have reached an agreement about how to share your time, you can go to court and present it there.

Courts use a standard called the "best interests analysis" to make custody decisions. The judge is supposed to look at each child's individual situation and make a decision based on what is right for that child. There is no preference given to birth parents over adoptive parents, and it does not matter who legally adopted a child first, if both parents adopted. If you are going to litigate custody, be prepared for mudslinging. Each parent tries to show that the other is not a good parent. In many states, the child's wishes are considered by the court when the child is mature enough to offer an opinion. In most states, this age is 12 or 13 years old, but it is decided on an individual basis.

Because court proceedings can get very unfriendly, it is a very good idea to try to reach an agreement first on your own. If you can't, you should see a mediator to help you come to a settlement.

Law Guardians/Guardians Ad Litem

In most states, when you file a custody petition in family court, even if you file a settlement agreement at the same time, the court appoints an attorney who is paid by the state to represent your child or children in the case. This person is called a law guardian or guardian ad litem (the name differs by state). He or she gets to know your child and the facts of your situation. Then either he or she makes a recommendation to the court about how the case should be decided, or he or she takes an active role and acts like a party in the case, calling witnesses and presenting evidence.

The law guardian can feel like an intrusion to you. Especially if you've filed papers just asking the court to approve your settlement, it can feel unnecessary to have someone else stick their nose in your business. However, there is no way to avoid this, so if a law guardian is assigned to your case, you need to be courteous to him or her. There's no guarantee you'll get a gay-friendly law guardian, but the law guardian's job should be only to look out for the best interest of your child. And if you've reached a settlement that works for both of you, it's unlikely the law guardian would protest. If you are going to trial, you can expect the law guardian to be more active and do home visits and interview you and your ex. It's always best to be honest with the law guardian. Remember, he or she wants just what you do—the best thing for your child. The following are some tips for dealing with a law guardian:

▼ Make your child available to him or her.

▼ Be courteous and respectful and try not to assume the worst.

▼ Be ready to open your home to him or her.

▼ If you are going to trial, be prepared to explain to him or her why you're right and your partner is wrong.

▼ Tell your child to speak honestly with him or her.

▼ Don't make your child promises or offer rewards linked to what he or she tells the law guardian.

Parenting Plans

A parenting plan is the schedule you will follow to share time with your child. It also often includes other agreements, such as how far in advance you will notify each other of schedule change requests or how you will introduce new partners to your child.

If you are both legal parents, you will need to prepare a written parenting plan that you will present to the court or to your lawyers. The plan must be approved by the court. When submitting a plan to the court make sure that it includes:

▼ An indication of how custody has been decided.

▼ What the parenting plan/visitation schedule is.

▼ A statement that parenting access/visitation will also occur at other times as agreed upon by the parties (this gives you the flexibility to make changes).

▼ A statement that says both parents shall have access to the child's medical and educational records (if this is something you both want).

If you are both legal parents, the first decision to make is custody. Joint legal custody means both of you have decision-making authority and must decide things about your child together. Sole legal custody means only one parent can make important decisions about the child. Physical custody describes where the child will be at different times. Some parents opt to use joint physical custody, which splits the child's time between them. Most parents however have arrangements where the child lives primarily at one parent's home and spends time with the other parent (often called visitation or access).

The parenting schedule can be anything that works for both of you, but it is important that you create a schedule that takes your child's needs into consideration. Your child needs to spend time with both of you, but he or she also needs to be able to do his or her activities and home-work and have a social life.

A very common schedule has the child with the non-custodial parent every other weekend, and one evening per week. You can choose any schedule that works for you though. Be sure to include a line in your agreement including visitation at other times as agreed upon, so that you can adjust the schedule as you see fit.

Most parents also create a plan that shares holidays. Some parents designate certain holidays to each parent, such as Christmas Eve to you and Christmas to your partner. Other parents alternate the holidays on a rotational basis, so you have your child for Thanksgiving this year, but not next year. Make up a list of the holidays you want to include in your schedule. Common days include: New Year's Day, Easter, Passover, Memorial Day, Fourth of July, Labor Day, Rosh Hashanah, Yom Kippur, Thanksgiving, Christmas Eve, Christmas Day, and Hanukah.

Your child's birthday (or adoption day) is another day you may want to share. Many parents also create a schedule that permits each parent a block of time with the child over the summer or school vacations to allow for traveling together.

Other important aspects of your parenting plan include additional agreements, such as decisions about who will provide transportation, how far in advance you will make scheduling requests, whether the child will continue to go to certain activities no matter whose house he or she is at, whether you will use each other as the first choice for babysitting, and whether you will consult with each other about buying large gifts.

Realize that any parenting plan you make will need to be flexible and there will come times where you may have to completely revamp it. Your child's needs will change as he or she ages. A schedule that works for a 1 year old is not going to work for a 13 year old. It's also important to realize that things are going to come up for both of you and you're both going to need to make changes and adjustments to the schedule from time to time. A parenting plan is not something written in stone. Instead it should be fluid and flexible and shift as your family changes.

Negotiation

Because custody decisions and cases are emotionally charged, it is almost always better if you can work out a settlement rather than having to air your dirty laundry in court. A custody battle leaves scars and it can be difficult to parent together after you've spent months (and thousands of dollars) on a court case that focuses on emphasizing the negatives about each other.

Mediation can be a very helpful resource if you are having a difficult time working out a parenting plan. If you're negotiating on your own, it is helpful to sit down and look at both of your schedules. Leave the big question of custody aside for a while and instead work on building a schedule for the next month, based on your schedules and your child's schedule. In many cases, a pattern begins to emerge that can help you see how you should decide custody and a long-term visitation plan.

Input From Your Child

It's important to give older children input into the schedule. Teens in particular are busy with sports, school activities, dating, work, and social events. If you go to court, you'll find that the courts seek input from children from about age 12 and up. It is essential that you and your child are clear on the fact that children don't get to make the decision (it's not fair to put that burden on them), but that their feelings and thoughts are important and will be considered in any decisions you make.

Legal Strategies

You may wish to consider legal action to obtain a legal right to visitation. In order to bring a case, you must first prove to a court that you have standing (or a legal right to bring a case). To do this, you need to prove that you were "in loco parentis" (filled a parental role in the child's life). This sounds as though it would be simple, but legally speaking, most courts will not grant standing to a nonlegal parent.

If you are both legal parents, your case will hinge on a best interests determination. To prove that you should have custody of your child, some things that will be important for you to show are:

▼ Your emotional bond or connection with the child.

▼ The amount of time you spend with the child in comparison to your partner.

▼ The decisions you usually make for your child.

▼ Activities you usually do with your child.

▼ Day-to-day care you normally provide.

▼ Your availability and schedule now, making you the person best able to care for your child.

▼ Your living situation, which is conducive to caring for a child.

▼   Your support system.

▼   Your health, which allows you to care for a
     child.

▼   The fact that you never say negative things
     to the child about the other parent.

▼   Your willingness to make sure the child has
     a relationship with the other parent.

It can also be very helpful to keep a parenting journal,
in which you record everything you do with your child
and any problems that occur with the other parent. You
may need to bring in witnesses who can say good things
about your parenting abilities and bad things about the
other parents' abilities. If your child has any special needs,
it will be important to have a doctor or educator come in
and testify about this so that the judge understands the
child's situation.

❖Tara gave birth to a son, Donald, and her
partner Connie adopted him soon after his birth.
They raised him together until they broke up recently. Tara had left her job when he was born
and stayed home with him full time, while Connie
continued with her job as a radio personality and
supported them both. Their break up was rough
and Tara was filled with anger and resentment.
She was sure that Donald should have no contact
with Connie. Connie believed strongly that she
should have custody and that Tara should have
no contact with Donald. Each eventually hired
an attorney and papers were filed in family court.
They were lucky enough to have two attorneys who
believed that when possible, settlement was always
better in family cases. Their attorneys encouraged
them to see a mediator. They finally were able to

continued on next page

agree on a mediator and attended several sessions. The mediator encouraged them to think about what kind of plan would work best for Donald and suggested they look at their own schedules and lives. She talked to them about how a child needs two parents and how those two parents need to work together and cooperate. She was able to get Tara and Connie to acknowledge that they both should have an important role in Donald's life and each admitted to herself that she had been using the custody issue to punish the other. With the mediator's help, they created a plan that had Donald live primarily with Tara and spend three weekday mornings and every Sunday overnight with Connie. They also agreed that they would each stay involved with Donald's school and activities. Their plan has been in place now for several months. Each reports that although there were some adjustments they had to make, they have found that the plan is working well for all of them.

Nonlegal Parents

If you are a nonlegal parent and want to continue to have a relationship with the child, your best avenue is to try and convince your former partner that the child deserves to have continued contact with you. Present options that are not intrusive or over the top. For example, if your former partner is not on board with having you involved with the child, suggesting that the child come stay at your house every other weekend is probably going to get you nowhere. Instead, start slowly with a suggestion that you take the child out to dinner or to the zoo and then gradually build from there. The key is to get your former partner to see that you and the child are attached to each other, and that your presence has a positive influence on the child. You also want to demonstrate to your former partner that being involved with the child does not mean you are involved in your partner's life.

You're at a definite disadvantage if you are the non-legal parent and want to continue to have a relationship with the child. Make sure the other parent understands your point of view. Make it clear that you understand that you have no legal right, but you love the child as if he or she were your own. Explain that all you want is to continue to spend time with the child and love him or her. Be clear that you are not trying to take the child away from the other parent or interfere in his or her parenting.

Legal Strategies

You may want to consider legal action to obtain a legal right to visitation. In order to bring a case, you must first prove to a court that you have standing (or a legal right to bring a case). To do this, you need to prove that you were "in loco parentis" (filled a parental role in the child's life). This sounds as though it would be simple, but legally speaking, most courts will not grant standing to a non legal parent. In *T.B. v. L.R.M.* in Pennsylvania, a court granted standing to a nonlegal lesbian mother whose partner gave birth to the child during their partnership. Courts in New York, California, Florida, and Tennessee have denied standing to same sex partners seeking custody or visitation.

One case currently moving through the legal system is the case of Lisa and Janet Jenkins-Miller. The couple lived in Vermont and had a civil union before their baby was born to Lisa. Janet did not adopt, believing that the civil union law made her a legal parent. The couple later split up, and Lisa returned to Virginia to file for custody there. Janet filed in Vermont. Lisa says she is now an "ex-lesbian" and is using Virginia's refusal to recognize civil unions to support her claim to custody. A Virginia court gave her full custody, but appeals are ongoing. The Vermont court has ruled that they are both legal parents and have equal rights to the child. The important lesson from this case is that even if you live in a state where you are both considered legal parents, you may not receive that same consideration in other states.

In a similar case, Denise Fairchild gave birth to a child that she and her partner Therese Leach parented. When they split up, they filed a parenting agreement with the Ohio court that gave them coparenting rights. The two are now in dispute and Denise wants the court to throw out the coparenting agreement saying it is invalid because Ohio has banned gay marriage.

Sandra Holtzman v. Elisbeth Knott is an older case (1995), but an important one where Wisconsin gave visitation rights to a nonbiological/nonlegal parent. The court in this case applied a test to determine whether or not a nonlegal parent should have parental rights. The court concluded she should if they lived in the same home, if the biological parent fostered or consented to a parent-child relationship, if the nonlegal parent took on parental obligations by providing financially and contributing to the child's education, and if the nonlegal parent bonded with the child and established a parent-child relationship. Most courts do not follow this reasoning, but it is an important first step for recognition of the rights of nonlegal emotional parents.

If you are the nonlegal parent, you have a tough row to hoe. If you are able to obtain standing and convince the court that you have acted as a parent and should have the right to seek custody or visitation, you then need to look at the factors listed under legal parenting in the previous section and try to prove as many of those as you can. You need to show the court that even though there isn't a piece of paper saying this child is yours, in all other ways the child is connected to you with a parent-child bond. Your case has to focus on what is best for the child, not on who has legal rights to the child.

❖Ryan had sole custody of his daughter, Cara, from his heterosexual marriage. His ex-wife was killed in a car accident soon after their divorce. Ryan and Logan had been together since Cara was 4 years old. Now at age 15 she thought of both of them as her parents. She and Logan often hiked together and he was the one she turned to for dating advice. Ryan had gone through some changes and went back to school to become a nurse, where he met someone else. He and Logan agreed to a trial separation while he worked out what he wanted. During this period, Cara would come over to Logan's apartment after school frequently. Ryan graduated from nursing school and got a job in another city. He planned to move himself and Cara there. Logan felt as though someone ripped his heart out. First to lose Ryan, then to lose Cara was more than he could bear. Logan felt angry that there was no way for him to get a court in his state Cara to come back and stay with Logan over school vacations and he stayed in touch with her by e-mail, Instant Messenger, and emergency dating crisis phone calls, but it really never was the same. When Cara went to college, she ended up 30

continued on next page

miles away from where Logan was living and he took her out to brunch every Sunday. When Cara got married several years later, her father walked her down the aisle, but Logan was right there in the front row.

Chapter 11

Child Support

Child support laws will apply to you and your partner if you are both legal parents of a child. There has been extensive litigation over this issue in many states and the decisions are clear—legal parents have a duty to support their children, even if they are not biological parents.

If one of you is a legal parent and the other is not, there is no legal obligation by the nonlegal parent to pay child support (unless you have won the right to custody or visitation—then the court will probably hold that you are a de facto parent and as such must support your child). However, the laws are different for couples living with domestic partnerships in California. If you are not a biological parent and have not adopted the child but the child was born to or adopted by your partner during your partnership, you are presumed to be responsible for child support under the domestic partnership law.

Understanding Child Support

Child support laws were put into place to ensure that children are supported by both parents and to prevent one parent from having to carry the entire financial burden involved in raising a child. Child support laws are not meant to punish noncustodial parents or reward custodial parents, but instead are supposed to make sure that the child has a reasonable lifestyle (it's supposed to be comparable to the lifestyle before the breakup) and his or her needs are met. Child support, however, does not have to be used for child-specific expenses, which surprises many people. There is no follow-up or requirements about how child support money must be spent by the parent receiving it.

When thinking about child support, it is important to keep the reason for it in mind and to focus on the benefit it provides to the child, and not how the two parents perceive it or feel about it. Child support laws do not make any distinction when it comes to a parents' sex or sexual persuasion. Child support can only be applied to parents that are on the birth certificate or have a custody order from a court.

Child support payments are not tax deductible by the parent making the payments and they do not count as income for the parent receiving them.

Types of Child Support

All states have child support laws that set a statutory amount that is based on the number of children in the family and the parents' incomes. There is a minimum child support requirement that applies even to indigent parents.

Child support laws also have provisions for educational and medical expenses. Parents can split these or one parent can be responsible. Child support laws also require one parent to provide health insurance for the child.

Other expenses you may want to discuss include:

▼ College tuition and college savings accounts.

▼ Allowances.

▼ Holiday and birthday gifts.

▼ Special occasions such as proms and graduations.

▼ First cars and auto insurance.

▼ Birthday parties.

▼ Weddings.

▼ Bar and bat mitzvahs, first communions, confirmations, or quinceñearas.

▼ Travel to and from parents' homes if it requires airfare, bus, or train fares.

▼ School/activities supplies and expenses such as field trips, club dues, books, school clothes, tutors, private lessons, costumes, photographs, registration fees, equipment, instruments, computers, and more.

In addition to discussing what expenses are to be paid, discuss *how* they will be paid. Some parents keep a running tally, assign a percent to each parent, and settle once a year. Others have one parent who pays all expenses for sports while the other pays all expenses for music. Another option is to assign expenses for specific things to each parent. You can create any arrangement that works for you.

Calculating Child Support

If you are the parent who will be paying child support, it will be mainly based on your income. Your income is adjusted for FICA and other deductions and then a percentage is applied to your income. This percent varies by state. In some states for example it is 17 percent for one child, 25 percent for two, 29 percent for three, 31 percent for four, and 35 percent for five or more. There is a minimum level of child support ($25 or $50 usually) that is applicable no matter how low the noncustodial parent's income is. You can calculate child support online using these state calculators: *www.alllaw.com/calculators/childsupport.*

Child support can be ordered by a divorce court or a family court. You don't have to get a legal divorce to have child support decided in court. Any family can go to family court and have child support handled. As with anything else, you can make your own decisions and settlements about child support (realizing that any transfer of funds done outside a court order could be considered taxable income or a gift, triggering gift tax), but if you go to court, your agreement must be approved by the court. That means it must either follow your state's percentages, or it must offer good reasons why you are deviating from those standards. If you plan on deviating from your state standards, it is important to have an attorney who can help frame your agreement in a way that will make it acceptable to the court.

Child support ends when the child reaches an age set by your state laws, usually 18, 19, 20, or 21 or when the child becomes emancipated (lives independently).

How Child Support Is Paid

Most parents arrange to pay child support weekly or twice a month. If you have your child support agreement approved by the court, you have the option of paying child support directly from one partner to the other, or the partner paying the support can pay it to the state child support enforcement bureau. The bureau tracks the payments, sends the money to the custodial parent, and handles enforcement proceedings if payment is not made.

❖Christopher and Raymond adopted a daughter from their state foster care system. When their relationship ended, they agreed that Raymond would have custody and Christopher would remain actively involved in her life. They got a family court order directing custody. After that was settled, a court employee asked them if they would next be determining child support. This was not something they had considered at all, although they had both just assumed they would continue to financially support her together. Raymond finally told Christopher that he did not feel he could file a child support case against him and could not legally seem to accuse him of not providing for their child. Christopher was touched that Raymond still trusted him in this respect but explained that he really wanted to pay child support and to have that legal responsibility for his child. Raymond filed the papers. Raymond earned $865 a week and Christopher earned $1,153 a week after deductions. The state rate for one child was 15 percent, so the court ordered that Christopher began paying $172 per week to Raymond. The two men also agreed that they would evenly share college costs. Christopher would continue to keep the child on his insurance plan and he would pay all co-pays and deductibles. The men agreed that payment would be made directly to Raymond because neither one wanted a state agency involved in their private business.

Choosing to Go to Court

If you get a legal divorce and are both legal parents, child support will be part of your settlement or court order.

You have no choice about that. If you are both legal parents of your child and you need to get a custody order, it makes sense to handle child support at the same time. But if you won't be going to court, maybe you don't need to. There's nothing that says you can't work out an informal child support arrangement, particularly if one of you is not a legal parent, but is an emotional parent. You do need to be careful because this kind of arrangement is not enforceable in any way and the money being paid could also be construed as taxable income by the recipient if it exceeds the gift cap of $11,000 per year.

Strategies

Hopefully, your divorce is an amicable one in which you are not having huge arguments over who gets what and who pays what. If you are in a situation where you can't agree and child support is one of the contested points, it may be wise to think about your strategy. If you are the parent who will be paying child support, your goal should be to minimize your income. The less you earn, the less you pay. You must provide an honest accounting to the court, but your goal should be to show as many expenses as possible. If you are the parent receiving child support, you want to be sure to show the court that the other parent earns more than he or she reports (this is particularly important if he or she is a business owner) and you will also want to put together an extensive list of your child's expenses, including medical care, prescriptions, school supplies, school clothes, sports equipment, musical instruments, uniforms, lessons and so on, to demonstrate how high your child's needs are.

While child support is a separate issue from property settlements, many couples look at them together and make some trade offs. When considering this is, it is important to remember that child support payments have a different tax effect (that is, they are not deductible by the paying parent or taxable to the receiving parent) whereas transfers of property or payments that are not technically child support may have a tax impact. The following are some tips for dealing with a child support case:

▼ Understand that child support cases are really financial calculations. There is some room for adjustment, but the outcome is primarily based on your state's formula.

▼ Remember that child support is not a punishment for the person paying it or a reward for the person receiving it.

▼ Keep in mind that child support is meant to provide a benefit for your child.

▼ Remember that lying on your financial disclosure form can subject you to perjury charges.

▼ Understand that child support cases are often heard not by a judge, but by a hearing officer or some other administrative official in the courthouse. The judge has supervision over the case and has to sign any order that comes out of the case.

Enforcement

If you have a child support order, it is important to understand how enforcement works. If the child support enforcement agency is receiving payments, they will handle enforcement. If not, the parent receiving it will need to file papers in family court if payment is not made. Non-payment can mean having your wages garnished, your income tax refunds held, your bank accounts attached, and your driver's license suspended. You can also be jailed for failure to pay child support.

Because the consequences are so serious, it is important to track child support payments. If you are the parent paying it, always get a receipt. If you are paying the state agency, keep track of the payments you make, check numbers, and date mailed. Doing this will not only help you remember to make payments, but will allow you to keep a record of payments so that if there is ever a question you will have a record.

If you are the parent receiving child support, keep track of when you are paid and what the amount is. This way if there is ever a missing payment you'll be able to pinpoint it right away.

Modification

Child support amounts are not set in stone and they can change. The most common reason for a modification is a change in the paying parent's income. If he or she gets a substantial raise or if he or she has a significant reduction in income, these can be reasons to ask the court for a modification of the amount of child support. A change in your parenting plan would be another reason for a change— if you went from your child primarily living with one of you to a situation where the child evenly splits time between your homes, this could lead to a change in child support.

It's important, however, to understand that child support isn't modified on a weekly basis based on how you spend time with your child. If a custodial parent went out of town on business for a week and the child spent that week with the noncustodial parent, child support would still be payable for that week. Also, if the custodial parent refuses to allow the noncustodial parent to spend time with the child or interferes with visitation, this is not a reason for not paying child support.

Other Financial Matters

Once you've determined custody and child support, you also need to think about tax exemptions. If you are both legal parents, each year, one of you can claim your child as a dependent on your taxes. You cannot both do so in the same year. Some parents alternate years, while others discuss this with their tax preparers and determine who stands to gain the most from taking the exemption. There is also the child care credit, for daycare expenses that only one of you can take each year.

Child Support Outside the Law

If you and your partner parented a child but were not both legal parents, there is no legal right to child support at this time. The nonlegal parent has no responsibility to support the child. This doesn't mean he or she can't continue to do so. There are several ways to implement a plan that will allow the non legal parent to support the child. The first option is to make payments to the legal parent, as if real child support were due. The issue with this is that it could be construed as taxable income for the custodial parent. If the yearly total passed $11,000, it would qualify for gift tax as well. The question you have to ask yourself is how traceable your transactions are going to be. If you're regularly receiving a check from your ex each week for $100, this is something the IRS may notice at some point. But if he or she hands you cash, there is no record of the transaction, and if you do not deposit the money into an account, but instead use it to buy groceries or clothes, it is likely no one will be the wiser.

Another option is to divide your property in a way that gives the custodial parent a greater share of the assets, giving him or her funds to support the child with. See Chapter 9 on property settlements for information on the tax consequences of this option.

The nonlegal parent could make payments to the child (to a Uniform Gift to Minors bank account for example), not exceeding $11,000 a year. This money could be earmarked for college expenses, and when combined with payments to the other parent (not exceeding $11,000 a year) could create adequate support.

The nonlegal parent can also pay for the child's education and medical expenses. If these expenses are paid directly to the school or medical care provider, they do qualify for gift tax, so a nonlegal parent could pick up all medical costs and pay private school tuition without any tax ramifications. It should also be noted that one parent can pay for the other's medical or educational expenses without tax consequences, freeing up the receiving parents own income to pay for other things.

If you do come to an agreement about child support, you need to consider whether you wish to write anything down. Doing so could create a contract and make this an enforceable agreement—good if you're the parent receiving payments, bad if you're the parent making them. Also a written agreement can be used as evidence for tax purposes, so that adds another layer of consideration.

> ❖Marina and Lois had raised a son together since the day Marina gave birth to him. Lois had never adopted him, but both had always acted as if she was his parent. When Lois and Marina split up, the child continued to live with Marina, but saw Lois on a regular basis. At the time their relationship
> *continued on the next page*

ended, Marina had a solid income as a car saleswoman and child support was not something they discussed, although Lois often took their son shopping for clothes, toys, and school supplies. A few years later, Marina was injured in an accident and unable to work for many months. Lois immediately began paying for their son's school costs to relieve Marina of that burden and began to bring groceries over every week. When Marina had used up her savings and couldn't make the mortgage payment, Lois paid it for her until she returned to work.

Caselaw

Courts are quite clear that when both parties in a same sex couple are both legal parents child support can be ordered. And in California, both parents are legal if the child is born during the partnership, regardless of whether an adoption has occured. However, things get murkier when legal parentage is not clear.

T.F. v. B.L. is a Massachusetts case where a woman agreed to have a baby with her partner, but left before the baby was born to her partner. The biological mother brought a case seeking to force the nonbiological mom to pay child support. The court held that no child support was due because the women had an unenforceable contract.

Kove v. Naumoff is an interesting Pennsylvania case in which one partner gave birth to five children using artificial insemination. They couple split up and the nonbiological parent sought custody and visitation even though she had never adopted the children. She won visitation and the court recognized her status as a parent. The biological mother then sued her for child support and she claimed she didn't owe any because she was not a biological parent.

The court held essentially that you can't have it both ways—either you're a parent and deserve to spend time with your kids and have the responsibility of supporting them, or you're not a parent at all and have no rights and obligations. The decision was important because it was the first time an appellate court ordered child support to be paid by a nonlegal parent.

Chapter 12

Spousal Support

Spousal support is a payment made from one spouse to the other to help him or her survive financially after the divorce or breakup. If you are in a state where your marriage is legal, you'll need to follow your state's requirements when it comes to spousal support (also sometimes called alimony). If you are not legally married and want to create some kind of spousal support plan, you need to consider your choices and the consequences.

Spousal Support After Marriage

In most situations, alimony is about helping one spouse become financially stable after a divorce, not about punishing or penalizing one of the spouses. Courts usually order alimony when:

▼ One spouse needs support while he or she gets an education, looks for a job, reenters the workforce, or makes a career change.

▼ One spouse is permanently disabled in some way.

▼ One spouse is elderly.

▼ There is a very significant difference between the spouse's incomes.

Courts usually limit alimony to one third the length of the marriage, although life long alimony is not uncommon for older or disabled spouses. Alimony can be payable in any intervals you agree on—weekly, bimonthly, monthly, annually, and so on.

Courts usually consider these factors when determining an amount for alimony:

▼ **The length of the marriage.** The longer you've been together, the longer the period of spousal support is likely to be.

▼ **Your health and your spouse's health.** If one spouse is ill or disabled, it is likely he or she will need financial support.

▼ **Your and your spouse's income and property.** If one of you is in a more difficult financial position, it is more likely alimony will be ordered.

▼ **You and your spouse's earning abilities, lost income, and workplace skills.** Often this is considered in regard to a spouse who stayed home to raise children or create a home for the couple and lost footing, earning ability or prominence at work to do so.

▼ **The contribution each partner made to the marriage.** This includes financial contributions as well as time spent raising children or supporting a spouse while he or she earned a degree or started a business.

▼ **The children's residence.** The spouse the children live with is likely to have greater financial needs.

▼ **How the spouses have treated the marital assets.** If one of you has withdrawn and spent all the money in a joint account, this would be a strike against that person.

▼ **Abuse.** If either spouse abused the other either physically or emotionally, it would have an impact on the type of award the court would make.

Alimony and Property

Consider spousal support hand-in-hand with your property settlement. There are plenty of trade-offs and negotiations involving these two issues. For example, you could decide to give one spouse a greater share of the investments, instead of creating an alimony agreement. Or you could decide to split assets equally but also set up alimony while one spouse works on reentering her career after years at home caring for the children. You could also decide that one spouse will pay off more of the couple's joint debt instead of paying alimony. Some couples also balance alimony with child support when creating a financial plan for the family.

❖Scot and Marcus lived together for two years and then registered their partnership under California's Domestic Partner Law. While they were together, Scot worked as a VP in a profitable ad agency. Marcus volunteered in many local organizations and was also an artist. When they ended their partnership, Marcus felt that he needed spousal support to help him get on his feet while he looked for a full time job. The court ordered spousal support, but based it on the length of their partnership from the date of

continued on next page

the registration of their partnership. Under California law, that is the only time period that can be considered. Marcus was happy to get some money, but kicked himself for not hurrying up and registering sooner.

Alimony and Taxes

Alimony is taxable income, meaning it is taxable by the person receiving it and tax deductible by the person paying it. When you're weighing property division against alimony, it's going to be absolutely essential that you look at the tax consequences of the options you are considering. Not only must you consider the fact that alimony is taxable income, but you also need to take into consideration the tax consequences of your property settlement. Your mediator may be able to walk you through some of these concerns, or he or she may recommend that an accountant evaluate your situation and come to a mediation session to discuss it with you.

Alimony as a Debt

It is also important to note that alimony cannot be discharged in bankruptcy. If one spouse owes alimony to the other and files for bankruptcy, alimony is not a debt that the bankruptcy court can wipe out, such as a credit card debt. Some people do not realize this and enter into alimony agreements, thinking they will go bankrupt and get out of having to make the payments.

Factors to Consider

Spousal support is normally not paid or received forever. You can create an agreement that terminates alimony in a variety of situations. Some you might want to consider are when:

▼ The person receiving it gets a degree or a job.

▼ The person receiving it cohabitates with someone else.

▼ The person receiving it earns more than a certain amount.

▼ The person paying it retires.

Alimony will automatically end when the person receiving it remarries (same sex marriages count as long as they are recognized by the state that issued your divorce or dissolution), or either party dies.

Understand that the length of alimony is uncertain. So if you're the one who is going to receive alimony, you might get all the scheduled monthly payments, or only one year's worth if the other person dies. However, a set sum or specific asset that you receive in the property settlement is certain—it's money you get today. When weighing alimony against an asset you receive outright, you're playing the odds. Getting $1,000 a month for three years versus $30,000 in cash up front is something to weigh. If you like the idea of regular payments but don't like the uncertainty of alimony, you can consider choosing an annuity for part of the property settlement instead of alimony, which brings more certainty.

Health Insurance and Expenses

When both of you have been receiving health insurance through one spouse's policy, you will need to make some decisions about coverage after the divorce. Options for the spouse who is not the policyholder include:

▼ Obtaining coverage through your own employer.

▼ Purchasing an individual policy.

▼ Exploring health insurance provided through a state program.

▼ Obtaining coverage through COBRA, a federal law that allows you to stay on your spouse's policy for 18 months after the divorce if one of you pays the cost of the premiums.

Health insurance and household expenses are items that one spouse may pay for the other during and/or after the divorce. It is important that you and your spouse examine the tax consequences of these options before making any decisions. It is extremely important that you are careful about categorizing these payments as alimony or property settlement, because there are different consequences for each. Remember that these expenses can be important bargaining chips.

Spousal Support if You Are Not Married

If you and your partner are not married or unioned in the eyes of your state, you can still create a spousal support plan, but you must be aware of the possible consequences.

The following are some tips on spousal support:

▼ Spousal support should be based around need, not emotional payback.

▼ Spousal support is part of an entire financial package that includes property settlement and child support.

▼ Think about both of your financial situations and try to create a plan that works for both of you.

▼ Realize that many couples do not create any kind of alimony plan—it is simply one option for your financial settlement.

Property Settlement

One way to help a spouse get on his or her feet financially is to give him or her a larger share of the assets you are dividing up. You have to be careful though. If you transfer assets from one spouse's name to the other, this is considered a gift for gift tax purposes. After you exceed the $11,000 cap per year, the value becomes taxable income. If you're transferring assets that were joint, you may run into this problem for half of the asset (assuming each partner owns half). It is also possible that a transfer of assets could be considered income.

Payments

If you decide one spouse will make payments to the other, you have to understand that this arrangement may not be enforceable (see later discussion on palimony) and that you also have to be aware of the gift tax law and the possibility that it could be considered taxable income. How you make payments is another important consideration. If your partner gives you monthly checks that you deposit in your bank account, this may be noticed by the IRS. But if he or she gives you cash that you use to buy things with directly, it is unlikely the transaction will be noticed. Note however that one person can pay another's medical or educational expenses directly to the school or health care provider without it being a trigger for gift tax or considered taxable income, so this is one area where you may be able to make support arrangements without worrying about consequences.

Negotiation Tips

If you're negotiating spousal support outside the reach of the law, it might be difficult to agree or determine what amount would be right. When you're thinking about and talking about alimony, the best way to go about deciding if you need to make some kind of arrangement is to prepare budgets for each of your new households and consider the property settlement you've reached. If you have children, also consider child support, if any. If one partner is going to be struggling financially, spousal support might be something you want to consider.

If you are the partner who is financially secure and you do not want to create any kind of spousal support arrangement, there is very little your partner can do, unless your partner can successfully prove a palimony case. (See later in this chapter.) There is no law compelling you to support him or her. If you don't want to argue about it, you might suggest that you would be willing to pay off some debt or give up some items of property just to resolve the whole issue once and for all.

If you are the partner in the lesser financial situation, you should consider all of your options. If you have children together and you have custody, you may want to seek child support and try to maximize your income from that. If your partner has ever promised to support you or take care of you, you might have a palimony case. You should also look at your property settlement creatively and find ways to maximize your benefits from that when possible.

Palimony

Palimony (sometimes called galimony when referring to gay couples) was first coined in the 1970s when the California case Marvin v. Marvin awarded a financial payment to an unmarried heterosexual life partner. Rhode Island upheld a galimony case in 2002 in *Doe v. Burkland*. Most states now have palimony caselaw. Palimony centers around a real or implied contract between the partners— a promise to support one another, usually when one partner stays home to care for the family or children and the other partner is the main breadwinner. You have no case for palimony unless you can prove that you and your partner had a contract or agreement about support and property sharing. If you are going to pursue a palimony case you will need an attorney who is experienced in handling these kinds of cases. Palimony cases can be hard to prove and generally are quite ugly. Palimony cases hinge on the judge and if you get a homophobic judge, he or she may be less likely to award palimony.

Health Insurance

If you are covered under your partner's health insurance plan, you are covered by COBRA (see earlier in this chapter for information) even though you are not married. You have the right to continue the insurance for yourself at cost for up to 18 months after your break up. If your partner pays the cost of maintaining the insurance for you, this may be considered income by the IRS.

❖Alex and Candy had two children and lived in a duplex that Alex had owned prior to their relationship. During their partnership, Candy stayed home and parented the children while Alex worked in the fashion industry. Alex felt a sense of responsibility towards Candy, but also knew she needed her freedom.

Alex was not sure how she could afford to pay child support and alimony and started to panic under the stress of it all. Candy was terrified of being out on the street with no job and two kids who would spend half their time with her.

continued on next page

The couple decided to go see a mediator who helped them take a hard look at their financial situation and each of their needs. They finally agreed that Candy did need some kind of support in addition to child support, but it was clear that finances were going to be tight for both of them. They decided that a good solution in their case would be for Candy to move onto the other floor of the duplex and pay a very low rent to Alex. Because the utility meters for the duplexes ran off the same meters, Alex would pay the full utility bills.

They agreed to do this for a year and then reassess where they were at. If Candy was able to become self-supporting, she would either move or begin to pay a higher rent and a portion of the utilities. If she was still having financial troubles, they would discuss if it was feasible to leave the status quo in place. Because Candy paid rent that was construed to be within the market range and her utilities were included, there was no tax consequence to her. Alex was still able to take deductions for repairs to the duplex because she was renting half of it to Candy. This arrangement also made it very easy for them to share time with their children.

Chapter 13

Mediation and Negotiation

In almost all instances, you're usually going to get through your break up more smoothly, more quickly, and with fewer problems if you can reach an agreement on your own. If you live in a state where you must get a legal divorce, you are still able to negotiate the terms of your settlement and then just have the court approve it. In other states you may have no option other than working things out yourselves if you want to avoid small claims court. This chapter will discuss how you can use mediation or one-on-one negotiation to reach an agreement that will work for both of you.

Mediation

An excellent option for couples who need some help in working through the divorce/breakup process, but who don't want to go to court (wisely) is mediation. Mediation is a flexible, empathetic, creative process that can help you and your spouse or partner reach a mutually agreeable resolution about the issues in your divorce or break up.

A mediator acts as a neutral third party who does not make decisions for you, but instead helps you find solutions yourselves. The emphasis in mediation is on compromise and fairness. Mediation gives you control over the issues that are important to you and allows you to reach an agreement that is custom fitted to your needs.

Benefits of Mediation

Mediation has many benefits. If you are in a relationship that is not recognized by your state, you have very few avenues available to you to resolve your divorce. Mediation services are available to all couples, no matter what sex they are.

Even if you do have the alternative of a court procedure, mediation is likely to cost less, because you will not need to pay your attorneys for court time. Mediation is a process where conflict is de-emphasized and cooperation is highlighted. The idea is that you entered into this relationship together and made decisions together about sharing your lives and finances. Because of this, it only makes sense that you should work together to make the decisions that will unravel that.

There are no time limits in mediation—you can resolve things as quickly or as slowly as you would prefer, at your own pace. Mediation is beneficial if you have children. The process takes into account the children's needs and helps you create a co-parenting relationship that will survive the end of your partnership. Mediation not only helps you resolve the disputes you have today, but it teaches you dispute resolution techniques so that you can resolve future problems together (and if you have children together or are going to have ongoing contact with each other, it is likely you will disagree again in the future).

Mediation is a flexible and creative process that allows you to talk about and consider anything you want. For example, while your state might not have laws giving you spousal support rights, in mediation, you can talk about and reach an agreement about this. Mediation empowers both participants and allows them to make the decisions about their own lives.

Basics of Mediation

Mediation is designed to be a process that puts the power into the hands of the couple. Your mediator is there as a guide only. He or she might point out alternatives you might not have considered, but he or she will not take sides, or make any decisions for you.

The mediator will remain completely neutral throughout the entire process, but he or she will provide you with legal information and resources when you need them. The mediator is also there as a neutral referee. Mediation is supposed to be a respectful process that encourages and allows turn-taking. Both participants should have opportunities to speak and offer possible resolutions. The mediation room is a safe place where name-calling or violence is not allowed. Participants also must be honest and completely disclose all of their financial information (this is required if you will be getting a legal divorce), so that everyone has the same information.

You choose your mediator, so you can be certain he or she is gay friendly, unlike when you go to court where you have to take whatever judge you are assigned. You and your partner can choose a mediator you are both comfortable with, and who understands your issues and concerns.

The mediator will keep your discussions and information confidential, although it is important to know that attorney-client privilege does not apply and the mediator could be compelled to testify about things discussed in mediation.

The mediator cannot give you personal legal advice, although he or she can provide legal information. Because of this, mediators will recommend that you and your partner see separate attorneys to get an idea of what kind of options and possibilities you would face if you decided to pursue your case in court. An attorney can point out what your rights are under your state's laws and your likelihood of succeeding. Because you only consult with outside attorneys and do not pay them to handle your case, mediation still costs less than having attorneys handle your case.

Mediation is not meant to be therapy where you talk about the origins of your problems and deal with emotional breakthroughs. It does, however, have a therapeutic aspect to it because you are working cooperatively with each other and making decisions that affect you both emotionally. Mediation is designed to allow room for emotions (unlike the court process) and the time to deal with them when necessary. However, overall, mediation is result-oriented—you are there to resolve some issues, not to heal your heart. Because mediation is so flexible you may be able to do things such as have ceremonies that officially end your relationship at a mediation session to allow you to obtain closure. (See Chapter 14 for more information about closure.)

Choosing a Mediator

Most mediators are either attorneys or therapists who have added mediation as a service they offer. Some have left their law or therapy practices to do only mediation. Both bring important skills to the process and the type of mediator you choose is a matter of personal preference.

There are also some mediators who are members of the clergy, accountants, or come from other professions.

There is no state or national licensing of mediators in the United States, so anyone can hang a shingle out and call himself or herself a mediator. Because of this it is important to look for a mediator who meets these qualifications:

▼ Minimum of 40 hours of divorce or family mediation training.

▼ Domestic violence mediation training or certification.

▼ Experience in handling gay or lesbian divorces/ break ups in your state.

▼ An understanding of the particular laws affecting your relationship.

▼ Membership in national, state, or local mediation organizations.

Different mediators use different techniques. For example:

Comediation: Two mediators work together, often a man and a woman, or an attorney and therapist.

Shuttle Mediation: You and your partner remain in separate rooms and the mediator goes back and forth between you. This is a good option if your situation is very volatile.

To find a mediator, you can contact your local bar association or local or state mediator's association for a referral. You can also contact the Association for Conflict Resolution *www.acrnet.com* or (202) 464-9700 for a referral. Area family law attorneys may also be able to provide you with a name. Your state family court may also maintain a list of mediators that participates in court referred mediation programs. You may be able to participate in one of the court referred programs (if your case would be one your state family court would hear), or simply contact one of the mediators on the list for private sessions.

Once you have the name of a mediator, schedule a free consultation. This will give you and your partner an opportunity to meet the mediator in person and get a feel for whether you are comfortable with him or her. It will also allow you to ask some questions, such as:

▼ What is your experience dealing with gay or lesbian couples?

▼ What kind of training do you have?

▼ What professional organizations do you belong to?

▼ What are your fees?

▼ Can I see a copy of the contract we would sign?

▼ In our case, what kind of written agreement would you prepare?

▼ How many sessions would you estimate our case would take?

▼ What mediation style do you use?

▼ What are your ground rules for mediation?

▼ Do you recommend we retain attorneys?

Costs

Mediators charge an hourly rate and usually require a refundable retainer to begin work on the case. Most mediators schedule one or two hour sessions every week or several times a month. The length of time it takes varies on a case-by-case basis. Mediators charge anywhere from $90 to $200 an hour, depending on their experience and the local going rate. You and your partner will be responsible for paying the mediator, but can divide that responsibility up however works best for you (your mediator can help you work this out). Many couples split the cost evenly, but if one partner has more financial resources, it may make more sense for him or her to pay the mediation costs.

Mediation Outcomes

The outcome of mediation is usually a written agreement. You have options with regard to this though. If you live in a state where there is a legal process to end your relationship, the mediator, or attorneys you hire, can prepare a settlement agreement, based on your mediation decisions, and file it with the court. If your mediator is an attorney, he or she may be able to prepare the actual document. If your mediator is not an attorney, a memorandum of agreement is prepared and sent to your attorneys, and the terms of your settlement are then just lifted out and placed into a legal document prepared by your attorney. If you use mediation, you may still need to make a court appearance to finalize your divorce, but you will not need a trial.

If marriage is not recognized in your state, mediation can still produce legal settlement agreements that can be filed with the court for custody and child support, if you are both legal parents of a child. Again, if your mediator is an attorney, the documents would be legal documents, but if your mediator is not, a memorandum of agreement would be prepared and the settlement terms would be lifted into a legal document by your attorney.

If your state has no recognition and you have no children, a written contract can be drawn up outlining the things you have agreed to in mediation. This may be legally enforceable in your state. You also have the option of completing mediation without a written agreement, if you feel it would impair your legal rights in your state. Some couples choose to draw up a written agreement, but do not sign it. This way they have something that is clearly defined and understandable that they both agree to honor, but they have not created legal obligations to each other that a court would get involved in.

Issues for Mediation

Because mediation is so very flexible, there really is no limit to the types of things you discuss or decide in mediation. You can work on big issues such as custody and property division, or you can talk about more esoteric issues such as how you'll keep the breakup from affecting your mutual friends.

Mediation can also help you decide what legal processes, if any, you will use to end your relationship. For example, if you have a Vermont civil union, but live in Nevada, you can discuss if it is important to either of you to obtain a Vermont divorce, or if you are content to simply go your separate ways and divide your property without a piece of paper from the state of Vermont. It is important that you and your partner take control of the mediation and use it to resolve the issues you need to work on. Your mediator is there to help you, not make decisions for you.

Later in this chapter you can read a complete list of issues commonly discussed in mediation or negotiation. In the meantime, here are a few tips for successful mediation.

▼ Come to all scheduled sessions and be on time.

▼ Try not to interrupt your partner when he or she is speaking.

▼ Provide complete financial disclosure, even if it is not required by your state.

▼ Be ready to approach problems in different ways and consider solutions that did not immediately occur to you.

▼ Be prepared to compromise.

▼ Remember that mediation is not about winning, but about resolving things in a mutually satisfactory way that allows you both to move on with your lives in a reasonable manner.

▼ Pay attention to suggestions your mediator makes. He or she is experienced in resolving these kinds of problems and may have some good ideas.

▼ Do not come to mediation with a set mind about what you will and will not agree to. You are there to negotiate and create an agreement that will benefit both of you.

▼ Be patient. It took you a long time to build your relationship and dissolving it cannot happen in one session.

❖Alissa and Janet lived in Vermont and had a civil union. When they broke up they knew that they had to go through the courts to end their union and determine child support and custody. Janet had heard about mediation as an option and she called her cousin who was an attorney to ask about it. He recommended that she contact the Vermont mediation association and get a few names. She did so and she called each one to ask a few questions. She asked what their fees were and if they had experience working with lesbian families. When she found one who charged a fee that seemed fair and who had worked with gay families, she and Alissa made an appointment. They went in for a free consultation. They explained the issues they needed to work through and some of the problems. The mediator showed them the agreement to

continued on next page

mediate that she used and explained her fees and retainer in detail. The mediator told them about her background as an attorney and the fact that she herself was gay. They discussed her mediation qualifications. Janet and Alissa felt comfortable with her and scheduled some sessions. They were able to complete mediation in two months and file a settlement agreement with the court, along with other required papers. Both felt satisfied with the process and were relieved they did not have to go to court.

Negotiation

Many couples find that they are able to negotiate the end of their relationship themselves. This works well for some couples, but can be a disaster for others. If you are going to try and work together, look at the following suggestions for some guidance:

▼ Lay some ground rules for your discussions.

▼ Ban offensive language, shouting, or emotional attacks.

▼ Schedule your meetings so you are both prepared for them and have time in your schedules to talk.

▼ Use a checklist (see later in this chapter) to help you navigate the issues you need to resolve.

▼ Take a break if you aren't making progress.

▼ Come to the meetings with all of the information you need at the ready (financial documents).

▼ Think about what you want and need before you meet.

▼ Take care of the no-brainers first, then move on to the more difficult issues. This will give you a sense of accomplishment and some momentum.

Checklist

It can be helpful to use a checklist such as the one below to help you move through the issues you need to resolve. This is a complete outline of all the issues that could possibly be facing a couple. Modify it to fit your situation by crossing out items that do not apply to you.

( ) Rules for Negotiation

Parenting Plan
( ) Decision-making (Sole, joint, divided)
( ) Living arrangements (Primary residence)
( ) Time-sharing schedule ("Regular schedule")
      ( ) Beginning and end, day and hour
      ( ) Notice
      ( ) Travel arrangements and cost
( ) Holidays
( ) Long weekends
( ) School breaks (February, Spring, Christmas)
( ) Summer vacation
( ) Birthdays (Children's, parents')
( ) Other special occasions (Mother's Day, Father's Day, and so on.)
( ) Other understandings

( ) Child care when ill
( ) Telephone access
( ) Gifts
( ) Travel (length of time, geographic location)
( ) Laundry
( ) Extended family ("grandparent's rights")
( ) Relocation
( ) Religion
( ) Decisions requiring mutual consultation
( ) Notification regarding illness, emergency authority
( ) Visiting if child is sick
( ) Access to records, notification of address and telephone numbers
( ) Provisions for review or modification
( ) Child(ren)'s voice in decision in marriage
( ) Sexual partners
( ) Dispute-resolving mechanism if you have future disagreements about parenting

Support
( ) Child Support
    ( ) Amount
    ( ) Time of payment
    ( ) Emancipation definition
    ( ) Escalation/reduction/suspension
( ) Child care costs
( ) Summer camp, lessons, special expenses
( ) School tuition
( ) College

( ) What is the child expected to do?

( ) What will parents do?

( ) What will be set aside now?

( ) Weddings, Bar Mitzvahs

( ) Spousal maintenance

    ( ) Amount

    ( ) Time of payment

    ( ) Duration

    ( ) Escalation/reduction/suspension

( ) Medical insurance (medical, dental, optical)

    ( ) Who provides for children, spouse

    ( ) Duration

    ( ) Access to records, notification

    ( ) Arrangements for submission to insur ance, reimbursement

( ) Unreimbursed medical, dental, orthodontia, and related expenses

( ) Life insurance

    ( ) Type

    ( ) Amount

    ( ) Duration

    ( ) Beneficiary arrangements

    ( ) Access to records, notification

( ) Disability insurance

( ) Provisions for disability, unemployment, and so on

( ) Need for financial planning for retirement, and so on

    Property

( ) Bank accounts

( ) Notes receivable

( ) Investments, stocks, bonds, mutual funds, tax shelters

( ) Marital residence
- ( ) Duration of occupancy
- ( ) Mortgage/rent obligations
- ( ) Taxes, insurance payments
- ( ) Repairs, "major repairs"
- ( ) Sale
    - ( ) Price
    - ( ) Division of Proceeds
    - ( ) Buy-out rights
    - ( ) Fixing up expenses

( ) Other real estate

( ) Retirement funds
- ( ) IRA, TSA, 401(K)
- ( ) Keogh plans (self-employed)
- ( ) Pension plans

( ) Business, partnerships interest

( ) Licenses and degrees

( ) Other assets (tax refunds due, patents, royalties, and so on)

( ) Personal property
- ( ) Cars
- ( ) Boats, RV's, and so on
- ( ) Jewelry, antiques, other items of large value

( ) Household items
- ( ) Division of items
- ( ) Provision for removal, storage

( ) Debts and loans
- ( ) Mortgage, home equity loans/lines
- ( ) Car loans

( ) Pets (ownership/residence, expense sharing, time sharing)

( ) Other property (gym memberships, frequent flyer miles, credit card points, and so on)

Other

( ) State income tax filings (for legally married couples only)

> ( ) How to file (joint, separately)
>
> ( ) Cooperation in filing, if joint; deductions, if separate
>
> ( ) Division of funds, assessments
>
> ( ) Prior year's joint returns refunds/assessments
>
> ( ) Dependency exemptions

( ) Future mediation fees

( ) Legal fees

( ) Estate rights waiver, need to revise wills

( ) Destruction/revocation of powers of attorney, hos pital visitation rights, funeral decision-making, and other documents created within the scope of the relationship

( ) How to proceed (immediate divorce, separation agreement, written agreement, oral agreement)

❖Tristan and Caleb had a big final fight and Caleb went to stay with his brother. He was there a few days, refusing to take calls from Tristan. "Dude, you've got to talk to him and get this worked out," his brother advised him. Caleb knew his brother was right so he went back to the apartment, but he and Tristan blew up again.

continued on next page

His brother nudged him again and this time Caleb sent Tristan a letter explaining what he wanted from the apartment and how he thought they should divide up the bank account. Tristan called and they agreed to meet and sit down and try to just sort out who got what without any big blow ups. Tristan's sister worked as a student services mediator at a local college and she told him that if they had any hope of working this out on their own that they needed to have a set agenda for what they had to decide and some ground rules to keep their anger in check. Tristan suggested this to Caleb and it worked. They followed the rules and had a uncomfortable moments as they expressed differing opinions, but in the end, were able to work out an agreement they were both satisfied with.

Working With a Friend

If you and your partner want to try to reach an agreement, but don't want to go to mediation or can't afford it and are finding that you just aren't able to negotiate one-on-one, asking a friend to help you may be a good solution. Choose someone you both are comfortable with and lay some ground rules out so everyone is clear on what will happen. Some examples include:

▼ The friend will listen non judgmentally to both of you, ask questions, and offer suggestions about ways he or she thinks you can resolve your dispute.

▼ You will meet at the friend's home because it is neutral territory.

▼ Your friend will meet with each of you individually then meet with you at the same time to discuss some possible solutions.

▼ Your friend will act only as a referee, making sure you both stay within the boundaries you've set up. He or she will not offer suggestions, but will assist in clearing up confusion between the two of ("John, I think what Mercer is saying is this...").

Chapter 14

Coping and Obtaining Closure

Coping with and getting over your divorce or breakup is probably one of the most difficult things you will ever face. Your entire world has changed and you've got to readjust your life plan, and make changes that affect your daily life as well as your long-term future. Dealing with all of this is not easy, but you will get through it.

Emotions Involved in Divorce

As you move through your divorce, you'll experience a whole host of emotions. What you're dealing with is an all-encompassing life change. It is a fundamental upheaval of who you are and where you're going. Living through this can be challenging. Understanding what to expect can help you get a grip on what you're going though. There are five basics stages most people move through as they cope with a divorce and it can be helpful to understand them. While this is a common path, it's not how everyone experiences divorce. If you don't find yourself going through these stages, or find that you go through them in a different order, or find yourself repeating them, it doesn't mean there's anything wrong with you.

Panic: Often the first thing people feel is panic and fear that their marriage or relationship is ending, or that their partner wants it to end. The long list of changes that the divorce will precipitate seems overwhelming at this point and people often believe there is no way they can cope with it. This is the "freaking out" stage.

Denial: It's completely natural and normal to go through a phase of denial in which you pretend as if there is nothing wrong, or through which you assume that you will get back together. In a way it is a defense mechanism that allows you to go on with life during a period when things are very confusing and upsetting.

Pain: At this point, the reality of what is happening sinks in and people often feel overwhelmed with sadness and hurt. A deep sense of loss is pervasive and debilitating. This is the point where many people feel a very deep depression and find that it is difficult to go on.

Anger: A natural step is to feel anger and rage at your partner and others. This is the point where you blame others for their role in what has gone wrong. Everything is magnified and missteps made by others can seem glaring and impossible to ignore. You're searching for reasons and ready to blame anyone.

Acceptance: The final stage is acceptance, where you accept where you are and what is happening. You feel ready to deal with whatever you need to do in order to move things along and get on with your life. This does not mean you are over it, but it does mean that you recognize that you can go on living and that the future might hold good things for you.

Coping

You shouldn't deal with all of this alone and you don't have to. What you are going through is a divorce, even if your state doesn't let you call it that, and a divorce is one of the biggest, most stressful life events you can ever face. You need people to talk to, shoulders to cry on, and distractions. Stick close to the people who understand what you're going through, and put some distance between yourself and those people who are not understanding or accepting.

If you feel as though it's all too much to handle, you should seek professional help. There's nothing shameful about finding a therapist who can help you work through the powerful emotions and life changes your divorce brings. Getting yourself mentally healthy and finding joy in life has to be a primary goal for you. Seeking out a therapist is not an admission that you're the crazy one or that the divorce is happening because of you. It's just a way to get some help and find some strategies that will make things easier for you.

To find a gay friendly therapist, contact: Gay and Lesbian International Therapist Search Engine *www.glitse.com*. Or call the Gay and Lesbian National Hotline at THE-888-GLNH.

Depression is common during breakups. Most people don't realize that depression is a real medical condition and there are treatments. Symptoms of depression include:

▼ Loss of energy and interest.

▼ Diminished ability to enjoy yourself.

▼ Decreased—or increased—sleeping or appetite.

▼ Difficulty in concentrating; indecisiveness; slowed or fuzzy thinking.

▼ Exaggerated feelings of sadness, hopelessness, or anxiety.

▼ Feelings of worthlessness.

▼ Recurring thoughts about death and suicide.

If you find you are experiencing symptoms of depression, or think you might be, see a mental health professional. You can also get information and help from the National Foundation for Depressive Illness at (800) 239-1295 or (800) 248-4344.

Finding Support

Everyone who goes through a divorce or breakup needs support. The best place to start is with family and friends. Lean on your loved ones during this difficult time and let them be there for you.

You can find advice, support, and discussion boards online at:

- ▼ *www.enotalone.com* (click on the gay and lesbian section).
- ▼ *www.gayhealth.com/templates/*
  1115658949513658958021
  /emotions?record=4&trycookie=1.
- ▼ *www.findarticles.com/p/articles/mi_m1589/*
  is_2000_Feb_1/ai_59086784.
- ▼ *www.goaffirmations.orghealth_services.asp.*
- ▼ *www.curvemag.com/speak/index.php.*
- ▼ *www.healthyplace.com.*
- ▼ *www.lgbtcenters.org/.*
- ▼ *www.danhazel.com*

You can find support groups in your local area by doing an online search or checking with your local gay community center or pride group.

Dealing With Those Who Don't Understand

It's no secret that lots of people don't "get" gay relationships, or are openly hostile about them. That is why it's difficult to marry, let alone get a divorce for gay couples. Some uninformed people think that gay relationships aren't as serious or committed as heterosexual relationships. If someone doesn't understand gay marriage, there's no way they are going to understand gay divorce with any kind of sensitivity. Aside from getting involved in activism, there are some things you can do to protect yourself from this kind of prejudice.

Always refer to what you're going through as a "divorce." This is what it is, whether your state recognizes that or not. So if an acquaintance asks why you're so down, don't explain that you and your partner broke up, instead say that you're going through a divorce. You will probably have to deal with "I didn't know you were married" comments, but you can explain that as far as you and your partner were concerned, you were in a committed marriage even if the state doesn't label it that way.

If acquaintances or coworkers are not understanding, you might want to spend five minutes explaining to them that what you are dealing with *is* a divorce in all aspects and is just as difficult as any heterosexual divorce. Changing minds one at a time may not be very efficient, but it can make a lot of difference in your circle of acquaintances.

If you find that the people you work with or know are not sympathetic or understanding in any way, your best bet is to ignore them. You know what you're going through, and how difficult it is. Their opinion does not change your personal and emotional struggle. It does not diminish it in any way, or make it less important. It's one thing to deal with ignorance and disdain when you are happily married or partnered, but it is another to deal with it when you are suffering. Your pain is real and if people can't respect that, then you may decide it is best to simply avoid those people.

Managing Financially After a Breakup

The emotional aspects of a breakup are difficult to face and work through, but in addition to these feelings and issues, you may be facing some financial difficulties, or at the very least, adjustments. You're going from two people living in one home to a single-parent family and dealing with less income than before.

A breakup can be financially devastating, particularly if you have children. The first thing you must do is look at how much income you will have, including any spousal or child support. Next take a look at what you have in terms of liquid assets. Then work out a budget that has your outgoing funds lower than your incoming funds. Easier said than done obviously. It may be helpful to consider:

▼ Getting a roommate or living with a friend temporarily.

▼ Drastically reducing expenses by canceling cable, moving to a smaller place, cutting your clothes expenses, putting a moratorium on new purchases, and so on.

▼ Looking for ways to supplement your income, through eBay sales, part-time work and so on.

▼ Limiting legal expenses as much as possible, or asking about payment plans.

▼ Creating a written budget and sticking to it.

▼ Asking for financial help from supportive family.

▼ Tapping into savings to get you through the first few difficult months until you get your feet on the ground.

In the months after the break up, the most you can hope for is to maintain your financial status quo. This is not a time when you can really think about getting ahead or making clear plans for the future. You need to concentrate on healing and trying to simply contain the bleeding from your savings as you struggle to find a new home (or afford your current one) and sort out all of your financial obligations. It's important to remember the positive side to this—you're moving forward to your own independent life where you and you alone will be managing your money. This is an opportunity for you to think about your future and find a new direction for yourself.

❖Darya was on her own after her marriage to Kate ended. They hadn't been married long and did not have a lot of joint assets or debts, which Darya supposed made things easier in some ways. However, because of the plans they had to start a family, Darya had reduced her hours at work and she had also contributed half of the deposit on the apartment. Darya and Kate had split the costs of the divorce half and half and Darya was now realizing that she was in a difficult financial spot. She had already moved to a small apartment of her own, but she was finding that, because of the emotional upheaval of the divorce, she was not really giving her finances the attention they needed. She decided to look for a different job

continued on next page

and became very focused on her career. She also made some lifestyle decisions and chose to discontinue her gym membership and take up hiking instead. She had always cooked elaborate meals for Kate, but now found she was happy eating simple things that didn't require a lot of thought or money. She also created a budget for herself and was able to keep her expenses in check. A year after the divorce she truly felt she had never been in a better place both personally, professionally, and financially. Although she still felt sadness and regret, she knew she had moved on and made a better life for herself.

Parenting After a Breakup

It may feel as though custody decisions, or making arrangements for a child to be part of both of your lives, is the tough part. The bad news is that it's going to get harder before it gets easier. Making those decisions and putting the arrangements in place is a very big hurdle, but actually living with it all can be a tough pill to swallow. Expect it to take at least one full year to adjust to the new arrangement with lots of ups and downs along the way. The good news is that you will be able to parent your child alone during your times with your child. Your children won't have to listen to arguments or be in the middle of conflict. Children of divorce do much better than everyone thinks, and your kids are going to be just fine.

Custodial Parent

If you are custodial parent, the one with whom your child lives most of the time, you might expect that the parenting plan arrangements you have made will not have that great of an effect on you. But you would be wrong. It is very difficult to be a custodial parent and give up enough control to allow your ex to spend time with and have a relationship with your child without you involved in any way. It is very tempting and very easy to try to insert yourself into the situation. The best plan is to force yourself to step aside and bite your tongue. Your child needs two parents and you have to allow him or her to have that.

Custodial parents often find they have a really hard time coping when their child is away with the other parent. Make plans and keep yourself busy. Remind yourself over and over that this schedule is good for your child.

It's also important to remember that just because you are the parent with whom your child spends the most time with, you are not the better parent, or the parent to whom your child is most attached. Your child needs both parents and loves both of you equally. Do not turn this into a competition or contest. The best thing you can do is to allow your child to know that you support his or her relationship with the other parent.

Noncustodial Parent

If your child does not live with you after the divorce, it is quite an adjustment to get used to seeing him or her only at times that are scheduled. The key to making it work is to stay in touch when you're not together—by phone, e-mail, Instant Messenger, and so on. When you are together try to do things together that are normal. Make dinner, watch TV, play in the yard, go to the library. Of course it's great to do special things once in a while, such as go to an amusement park or visit a museum, but the biggest trap most noncustodial parents fall into is trying to make up for what they think is lacking by showering the child with gifts or special activities. Just be yourself and spend normal time with your child. Your relationship will remain solid.

Treat the other parent with respect and consideration and help your child know that both of you are important parts of his or her life.

The Importance of Closure

Getting a divorce or ending your relationship is about more than dividing up the Limoges or figuring out how to share time with the dog. When you divorce, your world changes. You go from being part of a couple to being on your own. This can be a difficult transition and one you must face. Unfortunately, because gay marriage isn't recognized in most of the United States, there is a belief that when gay couples break up it somehow isn't as serious as a regular divorce. It's very important that you not let this kind of nonsense bother you. Your divorce is very real, and you know that.

To work through your divorce, you've not only got to deal with the practicalities of splitting your assets and the legalities of dissolving your union, but you must also find emotional closure for yourself. Getting to the point where you have closure can be a long journey and it is unreasonable to expect yourself to just get up and get over this. You must take some time to mourn the end of your partnership or marriage and then find a way to pick up the pieces and move forward. The best thing you can do is to have patience with yourself.

Ways to Work on Closure

One of the best ways to find emotional closure is to see a therapist who can help you work through all of your emotions and reactions. The bottom line is that you can't do this yourself and you need to lean on the people in your life who love and support you. When coping with a break up it is important to remind yourself that you are a good person and that just because this relationship did not work out, does not mean there is anything wrong with you, or that you do not deserve or will not find happiness.

When a relationship ends, you need time to adjust to the change in your lifestyle (such as if you have moved into a new place or are dealing with a visitation schedule), but you also need to get yourself together and do some new and fun things so that you can remember you are alive and you can enjoy yourself. It's normal to feel for a while as if you are going through the motions, but if you keep trying, you will eventually find that you can enjoy life again.

To help yourself work through closure, try the following tips:

▼ Put away photos or photo albums of you and your partner. This doesn't mean throw them out, but it does mean that you need to pack them away for now so that you don't have constant reminders every time you turn around.

▼ If you have stayed in the home you shared together, make some changes to make it feel different and fresh. Rearrange the furniture, buy a new bedspread, or move the elliptical machine out of the bedroom. Reclaim the space and organize it to fit your needs.

▼ Subtract your partner from the space. Maybe your spouse bought the leather club chairs or hung the art on the walls. Perhaps you spent a lot of time on the front porch swing. If it makes you think of him or her, get rid of it or put it away.

▼ Learn something new. Take a class, listen to a book on tape, experiment with a new sport, or try out a new hobby. You can grow and change, but you can only begin to do so if you take some time to find out where your interests lie. Learning something new will force you to concentrate and give you something to think about.

▼ Focus on you. So maybe you've always wanted a nice body, or perhaps you need to eat healthier. Now is the time to start a self-improvement kick. Physical exercise is a great way to clear your mind and get the endorphins going.

▼ Reassess who you are and where you're going. This is a good time to consider if you're happy in your job or if you want to move south. You've already had a big change roll through your life. Considering some other changes might give you the fresh start you crave.

Closure Ceremonies

Some couples find that they need something official to mark the end of their life together. If you and your ex can agree, a closure ceremony can give you both a feeling of tying up the loose ends and permission to move forward. You can have a closure ceremony anytime that suits you—when one of you moves out, when you complete mediation, when you divide up your belongings, when you get a divorce decree back in the mail, and so on.

There is no right or wrong way to have a closure ceremony—you've got to do what works for you in your situation.

The following are some suggestions for closure ceremonies to consider:

▼ Shaking each other's hands and simply wishing each other the best in the future.

▼ Hugging each other and saying thank you for the good times.

▼ Burning a copy of your written partnership agreement together.

▼ Doing a reverse unity candle ceremony. Light two separate candles from a large one and then blow out the large one together, signifying that you are now separate and not together.

▼ Taking a few moments to remember the fun you had together and promising each other you will try to remember that and not the bad times.

▼ Signing legal documents together.

▼ Dividing up photos.

❖Len and Justin chose to have a closure ceremony. When they had their commitment ceremony, because one is from the east coast and one is from the west coast, they had a sand unity ceremony. They each poured a jar of sand signifying their coast into a large vase until they were completely commingled. For their closure ceremony they divided the sand back into two jars. Friends thought it was a little sentimental and hokey, but for them it had meaning and gave them a sense of completion and full circle.

Post-Divorce Steps

After you officially end your relationship, there are some steps remaining for you to take to completely ensure a fresh start for yourself.

Your Will

If you have a will and you included your partner in it, it's time to get a new will drawn up. Be sure to destroy the old one, as well as any copies of it.

Power of Attorney

If you completed a form giving your partner the right to make financial decisions or complete financial transactions for you, you need to destroy the original and send letters to anyone you may have given copies to (such as banks, stockbrokers, real estate agents, and so on), and notify them that you are revoking it and ask that copies be returned to you.

Health Care Directive or Living Will

If you named your partner as your proxy for making health care decisions, or gave him or her the right to choose treatments for you, you need to destroy the original and ask for copies back from any medical care provider you gave them to. Have a new document drawn up listing someone else you trust with your health care decisions.

Hospital Visitation or Funeral Instructions

If you executed documents that gave your partner the right to see you in the hospital or make funeral decisions for you, you need to destroy this document as well as any copies.

Beneficiaries

If you listed your partner as a beneficiary on life insurance or a pension or retirement plan, you need to contact the company and revoke the beneficiary designation and name someone else.

Security

Change locks, passwords, usernames, access codes, and so on. Be sure that you have closed all joint accounts and credit cards.

Credit Report

Obtain a copy of your credit report after the divorce. You can obtain one free report from each credit reporting agency once per year (there are three main credit reporting agencies in the US) at *www.annualcreditreport.com*. Check the report for accounts that you have closed. If they are listed as still open, contact the creditors. Also look for unauthorized uses of your accounts or accounts opened in your name that you did not have anything to do with. Contact the credit reporting agency about these problems.

School and Health Care Permissions

If you are the legal parent of a child and your partner has no legal ties to the child, you may wish to revoke any permission you gave to schools or health care providers authorizing him or her to pick up your child from school, obtain medical care for the child, or attend school events. If your partner will remain an active part of your child's life, you might decide to leave these in place. This is a decision only you can make.

Name Changes

If one or both of you changed your names after you married or committed to each other, you may now wish to change your names once you are apart. If your state recognized marriages or civil unions, a name change will be part of your court order if you want one, so you don't need to take any other steps other than letting the court know you want to change your name.

If your state does not recognize your marriage or union and you want to change your name, you need to go through a simple court procedure. There are paralegal services that will handle the paperwork for you for a small fee, or you can handle it yourself. Usually it involves filing a petition with the court and then meeting a publication requirement (publishing the intended change in a newspaper in your area to alert creditors). If you wish to change your child's last name as well, you will need court approval and often need the consent of both legal parents.

Once you've taken whatever legal steps necessary to change your name, you'll want to make sure the change is noted on the following:

▼ Driver's license.
▼ Department of Motor Vehicles registrations and titles.
▼ Passport.
▼ Social Security Card.
▼ Bank accounts.
▼ ATM card.
▼ Investment accounts.
▼ Retirement accounts.
▼ Paychecks.
▼ Health insurance.

- ▼ Medical records/doctor's offices.
- ▼ Credit cards.
- ▼ Loans.
- ▼ Utility bills.
- ▼ Telephone company, so a listing will appear in your new (old) name in the phone book if you wish.
- ▼ Library card.
- ▼ Video rental card.
- ▼ Mortgage/home equity.
- ▼ Auto, home, and life insurance.
- ▼ Frequent flier miles.
- ▼ Gym and club memberships.
- ▼ Magazine and newspaper subscriptions.
- ▼ Internet/e-mail services.
- ▼ Store frequent shopper cards.
- ▼ Drycleaners and other local merchants with whom you have accounts.
- ▼ The post office, so mail with your new (old) name will be delivered.
- ▼ Your child's school and doctor's offices.

Appendix A

Support Information

Child Support

Child support calculators:
www.alllaw.com/calculators/childsupport
State child support laws and agencies:
www.acf.dhhs.gov/programs/cse/extinf.htm

Domestic Violence

www.rainbowdomesticviolence.itgo.com

Legal Help

The Center for Lesbian and Gay Civil Rights
1211 Chestnut Street, Suite 605
Philadelphia, PA 19107
215-731-1447
www.center4civilrights.org

GLAD Gay and Lesbian Advocates and Defenders
294 Washington Street, Suite 301
Boston, MA 02108
(617) 426-1350
www.glad.org

Human Rights Campaign (HRC)
919 18th St., N.W., Suite 800
Washington, DC 20006
(202) 628-4160
www.hrc.org

Lambda Legal
120 Wall Street, Suite 1500
New York, NY 10005-3904
(212) 809-8585 phone
(212) 809-0055 fax
www.lambdalegal.org

Mediation

Association for Conflict Resolution
www.acresolution.org or (202) 464-9700.

Support

National Association of Lesbian, Gay, Bisexual,
and Transgender Community Centers (NALGBTCC)
directory of local centers:
12832 Garden Grove Blvd., Suite A
Garden Grove, CA 92843

Websites

▼ *www.lgbtcenters.org*

▼ *www.buddybuddy.com/hertz-1.html*

▼ *www.gaytoday.badpuppy.com/garchive/people/082800pe.htm*

▼ *www.q-notes.com/bms4.htm*

▼ *www.enotalone.com*

▼ *http://www.gayhealth.com/templates/1115658949513658958021/emotions?record=4&trycookie=1*

▼ *http://www.dannhazel.com/Moving%20On%20Sample%20Chapter.html*

▼ *http://www.findarticles.com/p/articles mi_m1589/is_2000_Feb_1/ai_59086784*

▼ *http://www.goaffirmations.org/health_services.asp*

▼ *http://www.curvemag.com/speak/index.php*

▼ *http://www.healthyplace.com/communities/gender/site/comm_calender.htm*

Appendix B

State Specific Forms and Information

Massachusetts

Sample legal forms for divorce procedures can be downloaded from: *http://www.hampsireprobate.com/ Divorce%20Info/divorceinformation.htm.* These forms are samples only, however, they can give you a good idea of what to expect when beginning the divorce or separation process. The Website can also give you further information on the divorce process and ways of obtaining these forms and others.

TITLE III.

DOMESTIC RELATIONS

CHAPTER 208. DIVORCE

CAUSES FOR DIVORCE

Chapter 208: Section 1 General Provisions

Section 1. A divorce from the bond of matrimony may be adjudged for adultery, impotency, utter desertion continued for one year next prior to the filing of the complaint, gross and confirmed habits of intoxication caused by voluntary and excessive use of intoxicating liquor, opium, or other drugs, cruel and abusive treatment, or, if a spouse being of sufficient ability, grossly or want only and cruelly refuses or neglects to provide suitable support and maintenance for the other spouse, or for an irretrievable breakdown of the marriage as provided in sections one A and B; provided, however, that a divorce shall be adjudged although both parties have cause, and no defense upon recrimination shall be entertained by the court.

Chapter 208: Section 1A Irretrievable breakdown of marriage; commencement of action; complaint accompanied by statement and dissolution agreement; procedure

Section 1A. An action for divorce on the ground of an irretrievable breakdown of the marriage may be commenced with the filing of: (a) a petition signed by both joint petitioners or their attorneys; (b) a sworn affidavit that is either jointly or separately executed by the petitioners that an irretrievable breakdown of the marriage exists; and (c) a notarized separation agreement executed by the parties except as hereinafter set forth and no summons or answer shall be required. After a hearing on a separation agreement which has been presented to the court, the court shall, within 30 days of said hearing, make a finding as to whether or not an irretrievable breakdown of the marriage exists, and whether or not the agreement has made proper provisions for custody, for support and maintenance, for alimony, and for the disposition of marital property, where applicable. In making its finding, the court shall apply the provisions of section 34, except that the court shall make no inquiry into, nor consider any evidence of the individual marital fault of the parties. In the event the notarized separation agreement has not been filed at the time of the commencement of the action, it shall in any event be filed with the court within 90 days following the commencement of the said action.

If the finding is in the affirmative, the court shall approve the agreement and enter a judgment of divorce nisi. The agreement either shall be incorporated and merged into said judgment or by agreement of the parties, it shall be incorporated and not merged, but shall survive and remain as an independent contract. In the event that the court does not approve the agreement as executed or modified by agreement of the parties, said agreement shall become null and void and of no further effect between the parties; and the action shall be treated as dismissed, but without prejudice. Following approval of an agreement by the court, but prior to the entry of judgment nisi, said agreement may be modified in accordance with the foregoing provisions at any time by agreement of the parties and with the approval of the court, or by the court upon the petition of one of the parties after a showing of a substantial change of circumstances; and the agreement, as modified, shall continue as the order of the court.

A judgement 30 days from the time that the court has given its initial approval to a dissolution agreement of the parties which makes proper provisions for custody, support and maintenance, alimony, and for the disposition of marital property, where applicable, notwithstanding subsequent modification of said agreement, a judgment of divorce nisi shall be entered without further action by the parties.

Nothing in the foregoing shall prevent the court, at any time prior to the approval of the agreement by the court, from making temporary orders for custody, support and maintenance, or such other temporary orders as it deems appropriate, including referral of the parties and the children, if any, for marriage or family counseling.

Prior to the entry of judgment under this section, the petition may be withdrawn by mutual agreement of the parties.

An action commenced under this section shall be placed by the register of probate for the county in which the action is so commenced on a hearing list separate from that for all other actions for divorce brought under this chapter, and shall be given a speedy hearing on the dissolution agreement insofar as that is consistent with the wishes of the parties.

Chapter 208: Section 1B Irretrievable breakdown of marriage; commencement of action; waiting period; unaccompanied complaint; procedure

Section 1B. An action for divorce on the ground of an irretrievable breakdown of the marriage may be commenced by the filing of the complaint unaccompanied by the signed statement and dissolution agreement of the parties required in Section 1A.

No earlier than six months after the filing of the complaint, there shall be a hearing and the court may enter a judgment of divorce nisi if the court finds that there has existed, for the period following the filing of the complaint and up to the date of the hearing, a continuing irretrievable breakdown of the marriage.

Notwithstanding the foregoing, at the election of the court hereunder, the aforesaid six month period may be waived to allow the consolidation for the purposes of hearing a complaint commenced under this section with a complaint for divorce commenced by the opposing party under section one.

The filing of a complaint for divorce under this section shall not affect the ability of the defendant to obtain a hearing on a complaint for divorce filed under section one, even if the aforesaid six month period has not yet expired.

Said six month period shall be determined from the filing of a complaint for divorce. In the event that a complaint for divorce is commenced in accordance with the provisions of Section 1A or is for a cause set forth under section one, and said complaint is later amended to set forth the ground established in this section, the six month period herein set forth shall be computed from the date of the filing of said complaint.

As part of the entry of the judgment of divorce nisi, appropriate orders shall be made by the court with respect to custody, support and maintenance of children, and, in accordance with the provisions of section 34 for alimony and for the disposition of marital property.

Nothing in the foregoing shall prevent the court, at any time prior to judgment, from making temporary orders for custody, support and maintenance, or such other temporary orders as it deems appropriate, including referral of the parties and the children, if any, for marriage or family counseling.

Prior to the entry of judgment under this section, in the event that the parties file the statement and dissolution agreement as required under Setion 1A hereinabove, then said action for divorce shall proceed under said Section 1A.

Chapter 208: Section 4 Domicile of parties

Section 4. A divorce shall not, except as provided in the following section, be adjudged if the parties have never lived together as husband and wife in this commonwealth; nor for a cause which occurred in another jurisdiction, unless before such cause occurred the parties had lived together as husband and wife in this commonwealth, and one of them lived in this commonwealth at the time when the cause occurred.

Chapter 208: Section 8 Commencement of actions

Section 8. Actions for divorce in the probate courts shall be commenced in accordance with the Massachusetts Rules of Civil Procedure applicable to domestic relations procedure.

Chapter 208: Section 28 Children; care, custody, and maintenance; child support obligations; provisions for education and health insurance; parents convicted of first degree murder

Section 28. Upon a judgment for divorce, the court may make such judgment as it considers expedient relative to the care, custody and maintenance of the minor children of the parties and may determine with which of the parents the children or any of them shall remain or may award their custody to some third person if it seems expedient or for the benefit of the children. In determining the amount of the child support obligation or in approving the agreement of the parties, the court shall apply the child support guidelines promulgated by the chief justice for administration and management, and there shall be a rebuttable presumption that the amount of the order which would result from the application of the guidelines is the appropriate amount of child support to be ordered. If, after taking into consideration the best interests of the child, the court determines that a party has overcome such presumption, the court shall make specific written findings indicating the amount of the order that would result from application of the guidelines; that the guidelines amount would be unjust or inappropriate under the circumstances; the specific facts of the case which justify departure from the guidelines; and that such departure is consistent with the best interests of the child. Upon a complaint after a divorce, filed by either parent or by a next friend on behalf of the children after notice to both parents, the court may make a judgment modifying its earlier judgment as to the care and custody of the minor children of the parties provided that the court finds that a material and substantial change in the circumstances of the parties has occurred and the judgment of modification is necessary in the best interests of the children. In furtherance of the public policy that dependent children shall be maintained as completely as possible from the resources of their parents and upon a complaint filed after a judgment of divorce, orders of maintenance and for support of minor children shall be modified if there is an inconsistency between the amount of the existing order and the amount that would result from application of the child support guidelines promulgated by the chief justice for administration and management or if there is a need to provide for the health care coverage of the child. A modification to provide for the health care coverage of the child shall be entered whether or not a modification in the amount of child support is necessary. There shall be a rebuttable presumption that the amount of the order which would result from the application of the guidelines is the appropriate amount of child support to be ordered. If, after taking into consideration the best interests of the child, the court determines that a party has overcome such presumption, the court shall make specific written findings indicating the amount of the order that would result from application of the guidelines; that the guidelines amount would be unjust or inappropriate under the circumstances; the specific facts of the case which justify departure from the guidelines; and that such departure is consistent with the best interests of the child. The order shall be modified accordingly unless the inconsistency between the amount of the existing order and the amount of the order that would result from application of the guidelines is due to the fact that the amount of the existing order resulted from a rebuttal of the guidelines and that there has been no change in the circumstances which resulted in such rebuttal; provided, however, that even if the specific facts that justified departure from the guidelines upon entry of the existing order remain in effect, the order shall be modified in accordance with the guidelines unless the court finds that the guidelines amount would be unjust or inappropriate under the circumstances and that the existing order is consistent with the best interests of the child. A modification of child support may enter notwithstanding an agreement of the parents that has independent legal significance. If the IV-D agency as set forth in chapter 119A is responsible for enforcing a case, an order may also be modified in accordance with the procedures set out in section 3B of said chapter 119A. The court may make appropriate orders of maintenance, support and education of any child who has attained age 18 but who has not attained age 21 and who is domiciled in the home of a parent, and is principally dependent upon said parent for maintenance. The court may make appropriate orders of maintenance, support and education for any child who has attained age 21 but who has not attained age 23, if such child is domiciled in the home of a parent, and is principally dependent upon said parent for maintenance due to the enrollment of such child in an educational program, excluding educational costs beyond an undergraduate degree. When the court makes an order for maintenance or support of a child, said court shall determine whether the obligor under such order has health insurance or other health coverage on a group plan available to him through an employer or organization or has health insurance or other health coverage available to him at a reasonable cost that may be extended to cover the child for whom support is ordered. When said court has determined that the obligor has such insurance or coverage available to him, said court shall include in the support order a requirement that the obligor exercise the option of additional coverage in favor of the child or obtain coverage for the child.

When a court makes an order for maintenance or support, the court shall determine whether the obligor under such order is responsible for the maintenance or support of any other children of the obligor, even if a court order for such maintenance or support does not exist, or whether the obligor under such order is under a preexisting order for the maintenance or support of any other children from a previous marriage, or whether the obligor under such order is under a preexisting order for the maintenance or support of any other children born out of wedlock. If the court determines that such responsibility does, in fact, exist and that such obligor is fulfilling such responsibility such court shall take into consideration such responsibility in setting the amount to paid under the current order for maintenance or support.

No court shall make an order providing visitation rights to a parent who has been convicted of murder in the first degree of the other parent of the child who is the subject of the order, unless such child is of suitable age to signify his assent and assents to such order; provided, further, that until such order is issued, no person shall visit, with the child present, a parent who has been convicted of murder in the first degree of the other parent of the child without the consent of the child's custodian or legal guardian.

Chapter 208: Section 31 Custody of children; shared custody plans

Section 31. For the purposes of this section, the following words shall have the following meaning unless the context requires otherwise:

"Sole legal custody," one parent shall have the right and responsibility to make major decisions regarding the child's welfare including matters of education, medical care and emotional, moral and religious development.

"Shared legal custody," continued mutual responsibility and involvement by both parents in major decisions regarding the child's welfare including matters of education, medical care and emotional, moral and religious development.

"Sole physical custody," a child shall reside with and be under the supervision of one parent, subject to reasonable visitation by the other parent, unless the court determines that such visitation would not be in the best interest of the child.

"Shared physical custody," a child shall have periods of residing with and being under the supervision of each parent; provided, however, that physical custody shall be shared by the parents in such a way as to assure a child frequent and continued contact with both parents.

In making an order or judgment relative to the custody of children, the rights of the parents shall, in the absence of misconduct, be held to be equal, and the happiness and welfare of the children shall determine their custody. When considering the happiness and welfare of the child, the court shall consider whether or not the child's present or past living conditions adversely affect his physical, mental, moral or emotional health.

Upon the filing of an action in accordance with the provisions of this section, section 28 of this Chapter, or section 32 of Chapter 209 and until a judgment on the merits is rendered, absent emergency conditions, abuse or neglect, the parents shall have temporary shared legal custody of any minor child of the marriage; provided, however, that the judge may enter an order for temporary sole legal custody for one parent if written findings are made that such shared custody would not be in the best interest of the child. Nothing herein shall be construed to create any presumption of temporary shared physical custody.

In determining whether temporary shared legal custody would not be in the best interest of the child, the court shall consider all relevant facts including, but not limited to, whether any member of the family abuses alcohol or other drugs or has deserted the child and whether the parties have a history of being able and willing to cooperate in matters concerning the child.

If, despite the prior or current issuance of a restraining order against one parent pursuant to chapter 209A, the court orders shared legal or physical custody either as a temporary order or at a trial on the merits, the court shall provide written findings to support such shared custody order.

There shall be no presumption either in favor of or against shared legal or physical custody at the time of the trial on the merits, except as provided for in section 31A.

At the trial on the merits, if the issue of custody is contested and either party seeks shared legal or physical custody, the parties, jointly or individually, shall submit to the court at the trial a shared custody implementation plan setting forth the details of shared custody including, but not limited to, the child's education; the child's health care; procedures for resolving disputes between the parties with respect to child-raising decisions and duties; and the periods of time during which each party will have the child reside or visit with him, including holidays and vacations, or the procedure by which such periods of time shall be determined.

At the trial on the merits, the court shall consider the shared custody implementation plans submitted by the parties. The court may issue a shared legal and physical custody order and, in conjunction therewith, may accept the shared custody implementation plan submitted by either party or by the parties jointly or may issue a plan modifying the plan or plans submitted by the parties. The court may also reject the plan and issue a sole legal and physical custody award to either parent. A shared custody implementation plan issued or accepted by the court shall become part of the judgment in the action, together with any other appropriate custody orders and orders regarding the responsibility of the parties for the support of the child.

Provisions regarding shared custody contained in an agreement executed by the parties and submitted to the court for its approval that addresses the details of shared custody shall be deemed to constitute a shared custody implementation plan for purposes of this section.

An award of shared legal or physical custody shall not affect a parent's responsibility for child support. An order of shared custody shall not constitute grounds for modifying a support order absent demonstrated economic impact that is an otherwise sufficient basis warranting modification.

The entry of an order or judgment relative to the custody of minor children shall not negate or impede the ability of the non-custodial parent to have access to the academic, medical, hospital or other health records of the child, as he would have had if the custody order or judgment had not been entered; provided, however, that if a court has issued an order to vacate against the noncustodial parent or an order prohibiting the noncustodial parent from imposing any restraint upon the personal liberty of the other parent or if nondisclosure of the present or prior address of the child or a party is necessary to ensure the health, safety or welfare of such child or party, the court may order that any part of such record pertaining to such address shall not be disclosed to such non-custodial parent.

Where the parents have reached an agreement providing for the custody of the children, the court may enter an order in accordance with such agreement, unless specific findings are made by the court indicating that such an order would not be in the best interests of the children.

Chapter 208: Section 34 Alimony or assignment of estate; determination of amount; health insurance

Section 34. Upon divorce or upon a complaint in an action brought at any time after a divorce, whether such a divorce has been adjudged in this commonwealth or another jurisdiction, the court of the commonwealth, provided there is personal jurisdiction over both parties, may make a judgment for either of the parties to pay alimony to the other. In addition to or in lieu of a judgment to pay alimony, the court may assign to either husband or wife all or any part of the estate of the other, including but not limited to, all vested and nonvested benefits, rights and funds accrued during the marriage and which shall include, but not be limited to, retirement benefits, military retirement benefits if qualified under and to the extent provided by federal law, pension, profit-sharing, annuity, deferred compensation and insurance. In determining the amount of alimony, if any, to be paid, or in fixing the nature and value of the property, if any, to be so assigned, the court, after hearing the witnesses, if any, of each party, shall consider the length of the marriage, the conduct of the parties during the marriage, the age, health, station, occupation, amount and sources of income, vocational skills, employability, estate, liabilities and needs of each of the parties and the opportunity of each for future acquisition of capital assets and income. In fixing the nature and value of the property to be so assigned, the court shall also consider the present and future needs of the dependent children of the marriage. The court may also consider the contribution of each of the parties in the acquisition, preservation or appreciation in value of their respective estates and the contribution of each of the parties as a homemaker to the family unit. When the court makes an order for alimony on behalf of a spouse, said court shall determine whether the obligor under such order has health insurance or other health coverage available to him through an employer or organization or has health insurance or other health coverage available to him at reasonable cost that may be extended to cover the spouse for whom support is ordered. When said court has determined that the obligor has such insurance or coverage available to him, said court shall include in the support order a requirement that the obligor do one of the following: exercise the option of additional coverage in favor of the spouse, obtain coverage for the spouse, or reimburse the spouse for the cost of health insurance. In no event shall the order for alimony be reduced as a result of the obligor's cost for health insurance coverage for the spouse.

Vermont

Sample legal forms for divorce procedures can be downloaded from: *vermontjudiciary.org/courts/family/domestic.htm.*These forms are samples only, however, they can give you a good idea of what to expect when beginning the divorce or separation process. The Website can also give you further information on the divorce process and ways of obtaining these forms and others.

Title 15: Domestic Relations
Chapter 11: ANNULMENT AND DIVORCE
15 V.S.A. § 551. Grounds for divorce from bond of matrimony

§ 551. Grounds for divorce from bond of matrimony

A divorce from the bond of matrimony may be decreed:

(1) For adultery in either party;

(2) When either party is sentenced to confinement at hard labor in the state prison in this state for life, or for three years or more, and is actually confined at the time of the bringing of the libel; or when either party being without the state, receives a sentence for an equally long term of imprisonment by a competent court having jurisdiction as the result of a trial in any one of the other states of the United States, or in a federal court, or in any one of the territories, possessions or other courts subject to the jurisdiction of the United States, or in a foreign country granting a trial by jury, and is actually confined at the time of the bringing of the libel;

(3) For intolerable severity in either party;

(4) For wilful desertion or when either party has been absent for seven years and not heard of during that time;

(5) On complaint of either party when one spouse has sufficient pecuniary or physical ability to provide suitable maintenance for the other and, without cause, persistently refuses or neglects so to do;

(6) On the ground of incurable insanity of either party, as provided for in sections 631-637 of this title;

(7) When a married person has lived apart from his or her spouse for six consecutive months and the court finds that the resumption of marital relations is not reasonably probable.

§ 592. Residence

A complaint for divorce or annulment of marriage may be brought if either party to the marriage has resided within the state for a period of six months or more, but a divorce shall not be decreed for any cause, unless the plaintiff or the defendant has resided in the state one year next preceding the date of final hearing. Temporary absence from the state because of illness, employment without the state, service as a member of the armed forces of the United States, or other legitimate and bona fide cause, shall not affect the six months' period or the one year period specified in the preceding sentence, provided the person has otherwise retained residence in this state.

§ 656. Computation of parental support obligation

(a) Except in situations where there is shared or split physical custody, the total child support obligation shall be divided between the parents in proportion to their respective available incomes and the noncustodial parent shall be ordered to pay, in money, his or her share of the total support obligation to the custodial parent. The custodial parent shall be presumed to spend his or her share directly on the child.

(b) If the noncustodial parent's available income is less than the lowest income figure in the support guideline adopted under section 654 of this title or is less than the self-support reserve, the court shall use its discretion to determine support using the factors in section 659 of this title and shall require payment of a nominal support amount.

(c) If the noncustodial parent's available income is greater than the self-support reserve but payment of a child support order based on application of the guideline would reduce the noncustodial parent's income below the self-support reserve, the noncustodial parent's share of the total support obligation shall be presumed to be the difference between the self-support reserve and his or her available income. If the noncustodial parent owes arrears to the custodial parent, the court shall not order the payment of arrears in an amount that, by itself or in combination with the noncustodial parent's share of the total support obligation, would reduce the noncustodial parent's income below the self-support reserve, unless the custodial parent can show good cause why the payment of arrears should be ordered despite the fact that such an order would drop the noncustodial parent's income below the self-support reserve. Such arrears shall remain the responsibility of the noncustodial parent and be subject to repayment at a time when the noncustodial parent's income is above the self-support reserve.

(d) The court may use its discretion in determining child support in circumstances where combined available income exceeds the uppermost levels of the support guideline adopted under section 654 of this title.

§ 662. Income statements

(a) A party to a proceeding under this subchapter shall file an affidavit of income and assets which shall be in a form prescribed by the court administrator. Upon request of either party, or the court, the other party shall furnish information documenting the affidavit. The court may require a party who fails to comply with this section to pay an economic penalty to the other party.

(b) Failure to provide the information required under subsection (a) of this section shall create a presumption that the noncomplying parent's gross income is the greater of:

(1) 150 percent of the most recently available annual average covered wage for all employment as calculated by the department of employment and training; or

(2) the gross income indicated by the evidence.

§ 751. Property settlement

(a) Upon motion of either party to a proceeding under this chapter, the court shall settle the rights of the parties to their property, by including in its judgment provisions which equitably divide and assign the property. All property owned by either or both of the parties, however and whenever acquired, shall be subject to the jurisdiction of the court. Title to the property, whether in the names of the husband, the wife, both parties, or a nominee, shall be immaterial, except where equitable distribution can be made without disturbing separate property.

(b) In making a property settlement the court may consider all relevant factors, including but not limited to:

(1) the length of the marriage;

(2) the age and health of the parties;

(3) the occupation, source and amount of income of each of the parties;

(4) vocational skills and employability;

(5) the contribution by one spouse to the education, training, or increased earning power of the other;

(6) the value of all property interests, liabilities, and needs of each party;

(7) whether the property settlement is in lieu of or in addition to maintenance;

(8) the opportunity of each for future acquisition of capital assets and income;

(9) the desirability of awarding the family home or the right to live there for reasonable periods to the spouse having custody of the children;

(10) the party through whom the property was acquired;

(11) the contribution of each spouse in the acquisition, preservation, and depreciation or appreciation in value of the respective estates, including the nonmonetary contribution of a spouse as a homemaker; and

(12) the respective merits of the parties.

§ 752. Maintenance

(a) In an action under this chapter, the court may order either spouse to make maintenance payments, either rehabilitative or permanent in nature, to the other spouse if it finds that the spouse seeking maintenance:

(1) lacks sufficient income, property, or both, including property apportioned in accordance with section 751 of this title, to provide for his or her reasonable needs; and

(2) is unable to support himself or herself through appropriate employment at the standard of living established during the marriage or is the custodian of a child of the parties.

(b) The maintenance order shall be in such amounts and for such periods of time as the court deems just, after considering all relevant factors including, but not limited to:

(1) the financial resources of the party seeking maintenance, the property apportioned to the party, the party's ability to meet his or her needs independently, and the extent to which a provision for support of a child living with the party contains a sum for that party as custodian;

(2) the time and expense necessary to acquire sufficient education or training to enable the party seeking maintenance to find appropriate employment;

(3) the standard of living established during the marriage;

(4) the duration of the marriage;

(5) the age and the physical and emotional condition of each spouse;

(6) the ability of the spouse from whom maintenance is sought to meet his or her reasonable needs while meeting those of the spouse seeking maintenance; and

(7) inflation with relation to the cost of living.

§ 1206. Dissolution of civil unions

The family court shall have jurisdiction over all proceedings relating to the dissolution of civil unions. The dissolution of civil unions shall follow the same procedures and be subject to the same substantive rights and obligations that are involved in the dissolution of marriage in accordance with chapter 11 of this title, including any residency requirements.

Connecticut

Sample legal forms for divorce procedures can be downloaded from: *www.jud2state.ct.us/webforms/FAMILY*. These forms are samples only, however, they can give you a good idea of what to expect when beginning the divorce or separation process. The Website can also give you further information on the divorce process and ways of obtaining these forms and others.

Selected Laws:

Sec. 46b-40. (Formerly Sec. 46-32). Grounds for dissolution of marriage; legal separation; annulment. (a) A marriage is dissolved only by (1) the death of one of the parties or (2) a decree of annulment or dissolution of the marriage by a court of competent jurisdiction.

(b) An annulment shall be granted if the marriage is void or voidable under the laws of this state or of the state in which the marriage was performed.

(c) A decree of dissolution of a marriage or a decree of legal separation shall be granted upon a finding that one of the following causes has occurred: (1) The marriage has broken down irretrievably; (2) the parties have lived apart by reason of incompatibility for a continuous period of at least the 18 months immediately prior to the service of the complaint and that there is no reasonable prospect that they will be reconciled; (3) adultery; (4) fraudulent contract; (5) wilful desertion for one year with total neglect of duty; (6) seven years' absence, during all of which period the absent party has not been heard from; (7) habitual intemperance; (8) intolerable cruelty; (9) sentence to imprisonment for life or the commission of any infamous crime involving a violation of conjugal duty and punishable by imprisonment for a period in excess of one year; (10) legal confinement in a hospital or hospitals or other similar institution or institutions, because of mental illness, for at least an accumulated period totaling five years within the period of six years next preceding the date of the complaint.

(d) In an action for dissolution of a marriage or a legal separation on the ground of habitual intemperance, it shall be sufficient if the cause of action is proved to have existed until the time of the separation of the parties.

(e) In an action for dissolution of a marriage or a legal separation on the ground of wilful desertion for one year, with total neglect of duty, the furnishing of financial support shall not disprove total neglect of duty, in the absence of other evidence.

(f) For purposes of this section, "adultery" means voluntary sexual intercourse between a married person and a person other than such person's spouse.

Sec. 46b-44. (Formerly Sec. 46-35). Residency requirement. (a) A complaint for dissolution of a marriage or for legal separation may be filed at any time after either party has established residence in this state.

(b) Temporary relief pursuant to the complaint may be granted in accordance with sections 46b-56 and 46b-83 at any time after either party has established residence in this state.

(c) A decree dissolving a marriage or granting a legal separation may be entered if: (1) One of the parties to the marriage has been a resident of this state for at least the twelve months next preceding the date of the filing of the complaint or next preceding the date of the decree; or (2) one of the parties was domiciled in this state at the time of the marriage and returned to this state with the intention of permanently remaining before the filing of the complaint; or (3) the cause for the dissolution of the marriage arose after either party moved into this state.

(d) For the purposes of this section, any person who has served or is serving with the armed forces, as defined by section 27-103, or the merchant marine, and who was a resident of this state at the time of his or her entry shall be deemed to have continuously resided in this state during the time he or she has served or is serving with the armed forces or merchant marine.

Sec. 46b-45. (Formerly Sec. 46-36). Service and filing of complaint. (a) A proceeding for annulment, dissolution of marriage or legal separation shall be commenced by the service and filing of a complaint as in all other civil actions in the Superior Court for the judicial district in which one of the parties resides. The complaint may also be made by the Attorney General in a proceeding for annulment of a void marriage. The complaint shall be served on the other party.

Sec. 46b-51. (Formerly Sec. 46-48). Stipulation of parties and finding of irretrievable breakdown. (a) In any action for dissolution of marriage or legal separation the court shall make a finding that a marriage breakdown has occurred where (1) the parties, and not their attorneys, execute a written stipulation that their marriage has broken down irretrievably, or (2) both parties are physically present in court and stipulate that their marriage has broken down irretrievably and have submitted an agreement concerning the custody, care, education, visitation, maintenance or support of their children, if any, and concerning alimony and the disposition of property. The testimony of either party in support of that conclusion shall be sufficient.

(b) In any case in which the court finds, after hearing, that a cause enumerated in subsection (c) of section 46b-40 exists, the court shall enter a decree dissolving the marriage or granting a legal separation. In entering the decree, the court may either set forth the cause of action on which the decree is based or dissolve the marriage or grant a legal separation on the basis of irretrievable breakdown. In no case shall the decree granted be in favor of either party.

Sec. 46b-53a. Mediation program for persons filing for dissolution of marriage. Privileged communications. (a) A program of mediation services for persons filing for dissolution of marriage may be established in such judicial districts of the Superior Court as the Chief Court Administrator may designate. Mediation services shall address property, financial, child custody and visitation issues.

(b) All oral or written communications made by either party to the mediator or made between the parties in the presence of the mediator, while participating in the mediation program conducted pursuant to subsection (a) of this section, are privileged and inadmissible as evidence in any court proceedings unless the parties otherwise agree.

Sec. 46b-56. (Formerly Sec. 46-42). Superior Court orders re custody, care, therapy, counseling and drug and alcohol screening of minor children or parents in actions for dissolution of marriage, legal separation and annulment. Access to records of minor children by noncustodial parent. Parenting education program. (a) In any controversy before the Superior Court as to the custody or care of minor children, and at any time after the return day of any complaint under section 46b-45, the court may at any time make or modify any proper order regarding the education and support of the children and of care, custody and visitation if it has jurisdiction under the provisions of chapter 815p. Subject to the provisions of section 46b-56a, the court may assign the custody of any child to the parents jointly, to either parent or to a third party, according to its best judgment upon the facts of the case and subject to such conditions and limitations as it deems equitable. The court may also make any order granting the right of visitation of any child to a third party, including, but not limited to, grandparents.

(b) In making or modifying any order with respect to custody or visitation, the court shall (1) be guided by the best interests of the child, giving consideration to the wishes of the child if the child is of sufficient age and capable of forming an intelligent preference, provided in making the initial order the court may take into consideration the causes for dissolution of the marriage or legal separation if such causes are relevant in a determination of the best interests of the child, and (2) consider whether the party satisfactorily completed participation in a parenting education program established pursuant to section 46b-69b. Upon the issuance of any order assigning custody of the child to the Commissioner of Children and Families, or not later than 60 after the issuance of such order, the court shall make a determination whether the Department of Children and Families made reasonable efforts to keep the child with his or her parents prior to the issuance of such order and, if such efforts were not made, whether such reasonable efforts were not possible, taking into consideration the child's best interests, including the child's health and safety.

(c) In determining whether a child is in need of support and, if in need, the respective abilities of the parents to provide support, the court shall take into consideration all the factors enumerated in section 46b-84.

(d) When the court is not sitting, any judge of the court may make any order in the cause which the court might make under subsection (a) of this section, including orders of injunction, prior to any action in the cause by the court.

(e) A parent not granted custody of a minor child shall not be denied the right of access to the academic, medical, hospital or other health records of such minor child unless otherwise ordered by the court for good cause shown.

(f) Notwithstanding the provisions of subsection (b) of this section, when a motion for modification of custody or visitation is pending before the court or has been decided by the court and the investigation ordered by the court pursuant to section 46b-6 recommends psychiatric or psychological therapy for a child, and such therapy would, in the court's opinion, be in the best interests of the child and aid the child's response to a modification, the court may order such therapy and reserve judgment on the motion for modification.

(g) As part of a decision concerning custody or visitation, the court may order either parent or both of the parents and any child of such parents to participate in counseling and drug or alcohol screening, provided such participation is in the best interest of the child.

Sec. 46b-56a. Joint custody. Definition. Presumption. Conciliation. (a) For the purposes of this section, "joint custody" means an order awarding legal custody of the minor child to both parents, providing for joint decision-making by the parents and providing that physical custody shall be shared by the parents in such a way as to assure the child of continuing contact with both parents. The court may award joint legal custody without awarding joint physical custody where the parents have agreed to merely joint legal custody.

(b) There shall be a presumption, affecting the burden of proof, that joint custody is in the best interests of a minor child where the parents have agreed to an award of joint custody or so agree in open court at a hearing for the purpose of determining the custody of the minor child or children of the marriage. If the court declines to enter an order awarding joint custody pursuant to this subsection, the court shall state in its decision the reasons for denial of an award of joint custody.

(c) If only one parent seeks an order of joint custody upon a motion duly made, the court may order both parties to submit to conciliation at their own expense with the costs of such conciliation to be borne by the parties as the court directs according to each party's ability to pay.

Sec. 46b-56b. Presumption re best interest of child to be in custody of parent. In any dispute as to the custody of a minor child involving a parent and a nonparent, there shall be a presumption that it is in the best interest of the child to be in the custody of the parent, which presumption may be rebutted by showing that it would be detrimental to the child to permit the parent to have custody.

Sec. 46b-59. Court may grant right of visitation to any person. The Superior Court may grant the right of visitation with respect to any minor child or children to any person, upon an application of such person. Such order shall be according to the court's best judgment upon the facts of the case and subject to such conditions and limitations as it deems equitable, provided the grant of such visitation rights shall not be contingent upon any order of financial support by the court. In making, modifying or terminating such an order, the court shall be guided by the best interest of the child, giving consideration to the wishes of such child if he is of sufficient age and capable of forming an intelligent opinion. Visitation rights granted in accordance with this section shall not be deemed to have created parental rights in the person or persons to whom such visitation rights are granted. The grant of such visitation rights shall not prevent any court of competent jurisdiction from thereafter acting upon the custody of such child, the parental rights with respect to such child or the adoption of such child and any such court may include in its decree an order terminating such visitation rights.

Sec. 46b-69b. Parenting education program. (a) The Judicial Department shall establish a parenting education program for parties involved in any action before the Superior Court under section 46b-1, except actions brought under section 46b-15 and chapter 815t. For the purposes of this section, "parenting education program" means a course designed by the Judicial Department to educate persons, including unmarried parents, on the impact on children of the restructuring of families. The course shall include, but not be limited to, information on the developmental stages of children, adjustment of children to parental separation, dispute resolution and conflict management, guidelines for visitation, stress reduction in children and cooperative parenting.

(b) The court shall order any party to an action specified in subsection (a) of this section to participate in such program whenever a minor child is involved in such action unless (1) the parties agree, subject to the approval of the court, not to participate in such program, (2) the court, on motion, determines that participation is not deemed necessary, or (3) the parties select and participate in a comparable parenting education program. A family support magistrate may order parties involved in any action before the Family Support Magistrate Division to participate in such parenting education program, upon a finding that such participation is necessary and provided both parties are present when such order is issued. No party shall be required to participate in such program more than once. A party shall be deemed to have satisfactorily completed such program upon certification by the service provider of the program.

(c) The Judicial Department shall, by contract with service providers, make available the parenting education program and shall certify to the court the results of each party's participation in the program.

(d) Any person who is ordered to participate in a parenting education program shall pay directly to the service provider a participation fee, except that no person may be excluded from such program for inability to pay such fee. Any contract entered into between the Judicial Department and the service provider pursuant to subsection (c) of this section shall include a fee schedule and provisions requiring service providers to allow persons who are indigent or unable to pay to participate in such program and shall provide that all costs of such program shall be covered by the revenue generated from participants' fees. The total cost for such program shall not exceed two hundred dollars per person. Such amount shall be indexed annually to reflect the rate of inflation. The program shall not exceed a total of 10 hours.

(e) Any service provider under contract with the Judicial Department pursuant to this section shall provide safety and security for participants in the program, including victims of family violence.

Maine

Sample legal forms for divorce procedures can be downloaded from: *www.maine.gov/dhhs/bohodr/ terminmutualconsnt[1].doc.* These forms are samples only, however, they can give you a good idea of what to expect when beginning the divorce or separation process. The Website can also give you further information on the divorce process and ways of obtaining these forms and others.

Maine Public Law
CHAPTER 672
H.P. 1152 - L.D. 1579

Sec. 1. 15 MRSA §321, sub-§1

§2710. Domestic partner registry

4. Termination. A registered domestic partnership is terminated by the marriage of either registered domestic partner or by the filing with the registry of:

A. A notice under oath signed by both registered domestic partners before a notary that the registered domestic partners consent to the termination; or

B. A notice under oath from either registered domestic partner that the other registered domestic partner was served in hand with a notice of intent to terminate the partnership. If service in hand is not feasible, then substitute service may be accomplished in the same fashion as provided by the Maine Rules of Civil Procedure for commencement of a civil action. Termination under this paragraph is not effective until 60 days after service is complete.

5. Indemnity. If a 3rd party in reliance on the existence of a registered domestic partnership suffers loss because of a failure to receive adequate notice of termination under subsection 4, each registered domestic partner responsible for the failure to give notice is liable to pay the loss.

6. Forms. The registry shall develop standard forms for the declaration and termination of registered domestic partnerships.

New Jersey

Sample legal forms for divorce procedures can be downloaded from: *www.judiciary.state.nj.us/notices/reports/ todp040915.pdf.*. These forms are samples only, however, they can give you a good idea of what to expect when beginning the divorce or separation process. The Website can also give you further information on the divorce process and ways of obtaining these forms and others.

26:8A-5 Notice of termination of domestic partnerships to third parties; requirements.

_____5. a. A former domestic partner who has given a copy of the Certificate of Domestic Partnership to any third party to qualify for any benefit or right and whose receipt of that benefit or enjoyment of that right has not otherwise terminated, shall, upon termination of the domestic partnership, give or send to the third party, at the last known address of the third party, written notification that the domestic partnership has been terminated. A third party that suffers a loss as a result of failure by a domestic partner to provide this notice shall be entitled to seek recovery from the partner who was obligated to send the notice for any actual loss resulting thereby.

_____b._____Failure to provide notice to a third party, as required pursuant to this section, shall not delay or prevent the termination of the domestic partnership.

26:8A-6 Obligations of domestic partners.

_____6. a. The obligations that two people have to each other as a result of creating a domestic partnership shall be limited to the provisions of this act, and those provisions shall not diminish any right granted under any other provision of law.

_____b._____Upon the termination of a domestic partnership, the domestic partners, from that time forward, shall incur none of the obligations to each other as domestic partners that are created by this or any other act.

_____c._____A domestic partnership, civil union or reciprocal beneficiary relationship entered into outside of this State, which is valid under the laws of the jurisdiction under which the partnership was created, shall be valid in this State.

_____d._____Any health care or social services provider, employer, operator of a place of public accommodation, property owner or administrator, or other individual or entity may treat a person as a member of a domestic partnership, notwithstanding the absence of an Affidavit of Domestic Partnership filed pursuant to this act.

_____e._____Domestic partners may modify the rights and obligations to each other that are granted by this act in any valid contract between themselves, except for the requirements for a domestic partnership as set forth in section 4 of P.L.2003, c.246 (C.26:8A-4).

_____f._____Two adults who have not filed an Affidavit of Domestic Partnership shall be treated as domestic partners in an emergency medical situation for the purposes of allowing one adult to accompany the other adult who is ill or injured while the latter is being transported to a hospital, or to visit the other adult who is a hospital patient, on the same basis as a member of the latter's immediate family, if both persons, or one of the persons in the event that the other person is legally or medically incapacitated, advise the emergency care provider that the two persons have met the other requirements for establishing a domestic partnership as set forth in section 4 of P.L.2003, c.246 (C.26:8A-4); however, the provisions of this section shall not be construed to permit the two adults to be treated as domestic partners for any other purpose as provided in P.L.2003, c.246 (C.26:8A-1 et al.) prior to their having filed an Affidavit of Domestic Partnership.

_____g._____A domestic partner shall not be liable for the debts of the other partner contracted before establishment of the domestic partnership, or contracted by the other partner in his own name during the domestic partnership. The partner who contracts for the debt in his own name shall be liable to be sued separately in his own name, and any property belonging to that partner shall be liable to satisfy that debt in the same manner as if the partner had not entered into a domestic partnership.

26:8A-10 Jurisdiction of Superior Court relative to termination of domestic partnerships.

10. a. (1) The Superior Court shall have jurisdiction over all proceedings relating to the termination of a domestic partnership established pursuant to section 4 of P.L.2003, c.246 (C.26:8A-4), including the division and distribution of jointly held property. The fees for filing an action or proceeding for the termination of a domestic partnership shall be the same as those for filing an action or proceeding for divorce pursuant to N.J.S.22A:2-12.

____(2)____The termination of a domestic partnership may be adjudged for the following causes:

____(a)____voluntary sexual intercourse between a person who is in a domestic partnership and an individual other than the person's domestic partner as defined in section 3 of P.L.2003, c.246 (C.26:8A-3);

(b)   willful and continued desertion for a period of 12 or more consecutive months, which may be established by satisfactory proof that the parties have ceased to cohabit as domestic partners;

____(c)____extreme cruelty, which is defined as including any physical or mental cruelty that endangers the safety or health of the plaintiff or makes it improper or unreasonable to expect the plaintiff to continue to cohabit with the defendant; except that no complaint for termination shall be filed until after three months from the date of the last act of cruelty complained of in the complaint, but this provision shall not be held to apply to any counterclaim;

____(d)____separation, provided that the domestic partners have lived separate and apart in different habitations for a period of at least 18 or more consecutive months and there is no reasonable prospect of reconciliation; and provided further that, after the 18-month period, there shall be a presumption that there is no reasonable prospect of reconciliation;

_____(e)_____voluntarily induced addiction or habituation to any narcotic drug, as defined in the "New Jersey Controlled Dangerous Substances Act," P.L.1970, c. 226 (C.24:21-2) or the "Comprehensive Drug Reform Act of 1987," N.J.S.2C:35-1 et al., or habitual drunkenness for a period of 12 or more consecutive months subsequent to establishment of the domestic partnership and next preceding the filing of the complaint;

_____(f)_____institutionalization for mental illness for a period of 24 or more consecutive months subsequent to establishment of the domestic partnership and next preceding the filing of the complaint; or

_____(g)_____imprisonment of the defendant for 18 or more consecutive months after establishment of the domestic partnership, provided that where the action is not commenced until after the defendant's release, the parties have not resumed cohabitation following the imprisonment.

_____(3)_____In all such proceedings, the court shall in no event be required to effect an equitable distribution of property, either real or personal, which was legally and beneficially acquired by both domestic partners or either domestic partner during the domestic partnership.

_____(4)_____The court shall notify the State registrar of the termination of a domestic partnership pursuant to this subsection.

_____b._____In the case of two persons who are each 62 years of age or older and not of the same sex and have established a domestic partnership pursuant to section 4 of P.L.2003, c.246 (C.26:8A-4), the domestic partnership shall be deemed terminated if the two persons enter into a marriage with each other that is recognized by New Jersey law.

_____c._____The State registrar shall revise the records of domestic partnership provided for in section 9 of P.L.2003, c.246 (C.26:8A-9) to reflect the termination of a domestic partnership pursuant to this section.

Hawaii

Sample legal forms for divorce procedures can be downloaded from: *www.hawaii.gov/health/vita-records/vital-records/pdf/rbr_term.pdf.* These forms are samples only, however, they can give you a good idea of what to expect when beginning the divorce or separation process. The Website can also give you further information on the divorce process and ways of obtaining these forms and others.

Selected laws:

[§572C-7] Termination of reciprocal beneficiary relationship; filing fees and records; termination upon marriage. (a) Either party to a reciprocal beneficiary relationship may terminate the relationship by filing a signed notarized declaration of termination of reciprocal beneficiary relationship by either of the reciprocal beneficiaries with the director. For the filing of the declaration, the director shall collect a fee of $8, which shall be remitted to the director of finance for deposit into the general fund.

(b) Upon the payment of the fee, the director shall file the declaration and issue a certificate of termination of reciprocal beneficiary relationship to each party of the former relationship. The director shall maintain a record of each declaration and certificate of termination of reciprocal beneficiary relationship filed with or issued by the director.

(c) Any marriage license subsequently issued by the department to any individual registered as a reciprocal beneficiary shall automatically terminate the individual's existing reciprocal beneficiary relationship.

(d) If either party to a reciprocal beneficiary relationship enters into a legal marriage, the parties shall no longer have a reciprocal beneficiary relationship and shall no longer be entitled to the rights and benefits of reciprocal beneficiaries.

California

Sample legal forms for divorce procedures can be downloaded from: *www.ss.ca.gov/dregistry/forms/sf-dp_termbrochure.pdf.* These forms are samples only, however, they can give you a good idea of what to expect when beginning the divorce or separation process. The Website can also give you further information on the divorce process and ways of obtaining these forms and others.

CALIFORNIA CODES
FAMILY.CODE
SECTION 299-299.3

299. (a) A registered domestic partnership may be terminated without filing a proceeding for dissolution of domestic partnership by the filing of a Notice of Termination of Domestic Partnership with the Secretary of State pursuant to this section, provided that all of the following conditions exist at the time of the filing:

(1) The Notice of Termination of Domestic Partnership is signed by both registered domestic partners.

(2) There are no children of the relationship of the parties born before or after registration of the domestic partnership or adopted by the parties after registration of

the domestic partnership, and neither of the registered domestic partners, to their knowledge, is pregnant.

(3) The registered domestic partnership is not more than five years in duration.

(4) Neither party has any interest in real property wherever situated, with the exception of the lease of a residence occupied by either party which satisfies the following requirements:

(A) The lease does not include an option to purchase.

(B) The lease terminates within one year from the date of filing of the Notice of Termination of Domestic Partnership.

(5) There are no unpaid obligations in excess of the amount described in paragraph (6) of subdivision (a) of Section 2400, as adjusted by subdivision (b) of Section 2400, incurred by either or both of the parties after registration of the domestic partnership, excluding the amount of any unpaid obligation with respect to an automobile.

(6) The total fair market value of community property assets, excluding all encumbrances and automobiles, including any deferred compensation or retirement plan, is less than the amount described in paragraph (7) of subdivision (a) of Section 2400, as adjusted by subdivision (b) of Section 2400, and neither party has separate property assets, excluding all encumbrances and automobiles, in excess of that amount.

(7) The parties have executed an agreement setting forth the division of assets and the assumption of liabilities of the community property, and have executed any documents, title certificates, bills of sale, or other evidence of transfer necessary to effectuate the agreement.

(8) The parties waive any rights to support by the other domestic partner.

(9) The parties have read and understand a brochure prepared by the Secretary of State describing the requirements, nature, and effect of terminating a domestic partnership.

(10) Both parties desire that the domestic partnership be terminated. (b) The registered domestic partnership shall be terminated effective six months after the date of filing of the Notice of Termination of Domestic Partnership with the Secretary of State pursuant to this section, provided that neither party has, before that date, filed with the Secretary of State a notice of revocation of the termination of domestic partnership, in the form and content as shall be prescribed by the Secretary of State, and sent to the other party a copy of the notice of revocation by first-class mail, postage prepaid, at the other party's last known address. The effect of termination of a domestic partnership pursuant to this section shall be the same as, and shall be treated for all purposes as, the entry of a judgment of dissolution of a domestic partnership. (c) The termination of a domestic partnership pursuant tosubdivision (b) does not prejudice nor bar the rights of either of the parties to institute an action in the superior court to set asidethe termination for fraud, duress, mistake, or any other ground recognized at law or in equity. A court may set aside the termination of domestic partnership and declare the termination of the domestic partnership null and void upon proof that the parties did not meet the requirements of subdivision (a) at the time of the filing of the Notice of Termination of Domestic Partnership with the Secretary of State.

(d) The superior courts shall have jurisdiction over all proceedings relating to the dissolution of domestic partnerships, nullity of domestic partnerships, and legal separation of partners in a domestic partnership. The dissolution of a domestic partnership, nullity of a domestic partnership, and legal separation of partners in a domestic partnership shall follow the same procedures, and the partners shall possess the same rights, protections, and benefits, and be subject to the same responsibilities, obligations, and duties, as apply to the dissolution of marriage, nullity of marriage, and legal separation of spouses in a marriage, respectively, except as provided in subdivision (a), and except that, in accordance with the consent acknowledged by domestic partners in the Declaration of Domestic Partnership form, proceedings for dissolution, nullity, or legal separation of a domestic partnership registered in this state may be filed in the superior courts of this state even if neither domestic partner is a resident of, or maintains a domicile in, the state at the time the proceedings are filed.

Appendix C

Bachelor, Dina. *Break Up or Break Through*. Los Angeles: Alyson Books, 2001.

Boland, Mary L. *Your Right to Child Custody, Visitation, and Support*. Naperville, Ill.: Sourcebooks, 2004.

Hall, Marny. *The Lesbian Love Companion: How to Survive Everything From Heartthrob to Heartbreak*. San Francisco: HarperSanFrancisco, 1998.

Hazel, Dann. *Moving On: The Gay Man's Guide for Cop ing When a Relationship Ends*. New York: Kensington Press, 1999.

Isensee, Rik. *Love Between Men: Enhancing Intimacy and Resolving Conflicts in Gay Relationships*. Lincoln, Nebr.: Backinprint, 2005.

Pace, Anita L. *Write From the Heart: Lesbians Healing From Heartache*. Beaverton, Ore.: Baby Steps Press, 1996.

Pimental-Habib, Dr. Richard L. *The Power of a Partner: Creating and Maintaining Healthy Gay and Lesbian Relationship*. Los Angeles: Alyson Books, 2002.

McWhorter Sember, Brette. *Gay & Lesbian Legal Rights: A Guide for GLBT Singles, Couples, and Families.* Naperville, Ill: Sourcebooks., 2006.

————. *No-Fight Divorce: Save Time, Money and Conflict Using Mediation.* New York: McGraw-Hill, 2005.

Index

About the Author

Brette McWhorter Sember is a former family and divorce attorney and mediator who practiced law in New York state. She is the author of over 20 books, including *Gay & Lesbian Legal Rights: A Guide for GLBT Singles, Couples, and Families; Gay Parenting Choices: From Adopting a Surrogate to Choosing the Perfect Father; The Divorce Organizer Planner; No-Fight Divorce: Spend Less Money, Save Time, and Avoid Conflict Using Mediation;* and *How to Parent with Your Ex: Working Together in Your Child's Best Interest.* Sember is a member of The American Society of Journalists and Authors (ASJA), the New York State Bar Association, and The New York State Council on Divorce Mediation. You can find out more on her Website at *www.BretteSember.com.*